Smart
Chefs
Stay
Slim

Smart Chefs Stay Slim

LESSONS *in* EATING
and LIVING
from AMERICA'S
BEST CHEFS

Allison Adato

Foreword by Art Smith

 NEW AMERICAN LIBRARY

New American Library
Published by New American Library, a division of
Penguin Group (USA) Inc., 375 Hudson Street,
New York, New York 10014, USA
Penguin Group (Canada), 90 Eglinton Avenue East, Suite 700, Toronto,
Ontario M4P 2Y3, Canada (a division of Pearson Penguin Canada Inc.)
Penguin Books Ltd., 80 Strand, London WC2R 0RL, England
Penguin Ireland, 25 St. Stephen's Green, Dublin 2,
Ireland (a division of Penguin Books Ltd.)
Penguin Group (Australia), 250 Camberwell Road, Camberwell, Victoria 3124,
Australia (a division of Pearson Australia Group Pty. Ltd.)
Penguin Books India Pvt. Ltd., 11 Community Centre, Panchsheel Park,
New Delhi - 110 017, India
Penguin Group (NZ), 67 Apollo Drive, Rosedale, Auckland 0632,
New Zealand (a division of Pearson New Zealand Ltd.)
Penguin Books (South Africa) (Pty.) Ltd., 24 Sturdee Avenue,
Rosebank, Johannesburg 2196, South Africa

Penguin Books Ltd., Registered Offices:
80 Strand, London WC2R 0RL, England

First published by New American Library,
a division of Penguin Group (USA) Inc.

First Printing, April 2012
10 9 8 7 6 5 4 3 2 1

 REGISTERED TRADEMARK—MARCA REGISTRADA

LIBRARY OF CONGRESS CATALOGING-IN-PUBLICATION DATA:
Adato, Allison.
Smart chefs stay slim: lessons in eating and living from America's best chefs/Allison Adato;
foreword by Art Smith.
p. cm.
Includes index.
ISBN 978-0-451-23585-5
1. Diet. 2. Cooking. 3. Celebrity chefs—Health and hygiene—United States. I. Title.
RA784.A318 2012
613.2—dc23   2011045548

Set in Bembo Std
Designed by Pauline Neuwirth

Printed in the United States of America

PUBLISHER'S NOTE
The recipes contained in this book are to be followed exactly as written. The publisher is not responsible for your specific health or allergy needs that may require medical supervision. The publisher is not responsible for any adverse reactions to the recipes contained in this book.

While the author has made every effort to provide accurate telephone numbers and Internet
addresses at the time of publication, neither the publisher nor the author assumes any responsibility
for errors, or for changes that occur after publication. Further, publisher does not have any control
over and does not assume any responsibility for author or third-party Web sites or their content.

CONTENTS

For Julian and David,
my salt and pepper

FOREWORD

I N MY YEARS as a chef, I've made dirty rice for the Dalai Lama, Hummingbird cake for Lady Gaga, chicken with pomegranate sauce for the first George Bush, and a Valentine's Day dinner for Barack and Michelle Obama. I prepared countless meals for Oprah Winfrey as her personal chef and served my fried chicken to ballrooms full of Hollywood luminaries—and let me tell you, I'm not being proud when I say that they loved me for it. Everybody loves a chef, because everybody loves food.

But the most important meal I ever cooked wasn't for any of these big names. It was for just me.

It was a bowl of oatmeal with berries, and some egg whites scrambled with zucchini. The first time I ate that breakfast I weighed 325 pounds and had recently been given a diagnosis of diabetes, the disease that would take my father from me too soon. I knew I had to make changes, but even though I'd expertly prepared thousands of meals for other people—many tailored to their diet specifications—I had never given much thought to how to feed myself in a healthful way. If the boss said, "Art, I need steamed vegetables; I need a grilled piece of fish," that's what I gave them. But I never actually connected the good choices I was helping them make, with how I could improve my own poor habits. I knew other chefs who struggled with their weight, and some chefs who stayed fit—I just didn't know how the second group managed it, since *all* the chefs I knew seemed just as passionate about great food as I was, and still am.

Someone, in my case a health coach, needed to say, "Art, eat oatmeal. Eat berries. Eat egg whites and vegetables." So I did. Now, more than one hundred pounds lighter, I still have that same breakfast virtually every day. I've run marathons and in 2010 married my love, Jesus Salgueiro, wearing a suit that was smaller than the one I wore for my high school graduation.

The moral of the story is that while the motivation had to come from within, I still needed some inspiration from outside. That's what I hope this book will do: inspire you. When I heard that Allison planned to tackle the very question I once puzzled over, I decided right away I wanted to be part of this project, and share what I now know to be true: that you can be fit *and* enjoy wonderful food.

Maybe you want to lose a lot of weight and get healthy, and my story will speak to you. Maybe you're already on a path of eating well, but want to know how to do it with more flavor and flair. You might just be curious how some really fine chefs who are surrounded by food all day manage to make any peace with it at all. It isn't easy, and the way I went about it might not be for everybody. But what about the way Eric Ripert keeps fit by walking? Or how Michelle Bernstein finds ways to eat her vegetables while working long hours at Michy's? Or how Jacques Torres keeps off the weight he lost, and still eats a little bit of chocolate each day? When it comes to eating, I think Allison hit it right when she noticed people would rather take advice from folks who wear chef whites than white lab coats.

At this moment chefs in America, particularly those fortunate enough to be embraced by the public as celebrities, have enormous influence. I've tried to use mine responsibly, co-founding a charity, Common Threads, to teach kids from low-income families how to cook wholesome meals, with the goal of preventing childhood obesity.

But there's also a much louder message coming from the food media, celebrating butter and bacon and excess. This book represents an opportunity to say, "Hey, we don't all eat like that!"

There's a lot of collected wisdom here from my colleagues, who are among the best chefs cooking today. As I told Allison over a long-ago lunch at Art and Soul, in the end, it's about finding your happy—the thing that works best for you. It might be preparing a beautiful, healthful meal that you share with loved ones. It could be making smarter choices when you go to your favorite restaurant. Or it might be starting your day with a bowl of oatmeal and berries that you make just for yourself.

I hope that in these pages you find your happy.

Art Smith

WHY ASK CHEFS?

I'VE ALWAYS BEEN enchanted by restaurants. Don't mistake this to mean that my parents were not both great home cooks; they were. My mom somehow struck a balance between trying the latest 1970s California bean-sprouty health food trends and feeding us soul-warming briskets, stuffed cabbage, and latkes. My father, meanwhile, mastered a tight rotation of signature dishes like Turkish Pizza-pie Eggs, an anytime breakfast that he—and only he—still makes when we get together.

But restaurants were a big deal in my family. My mother's father, a Levy's Bakery truck driver and later a union leader, was hardly a man of means. Yet when we visited him he took the whole family to Windows on the World, the restaurant on the hundred-and-seventh story of the World Trade Center, where, above the clouds and New York City, my little brother had to wear a tie and we ate duck and clams (my brother spit one out in his napkin, which a waiter whisked away) and ice-cream sundaes. On another day Grandpa took us to an Italian seafood house on Long Island Sound that could be reached only by boat. In retrospect, I realize that must have been part of his restaurant hyperbole; there had to have been roads. But we went by boat and it was a wonder to a car-bound L.A. kid.

My grandfather would also tell stories of his Ukraine-born mother, an amazing cook who rolled her own paper-thin strudel dough at home and worked in the kitchen of a Lower East Side Italian place. I'm sure I romanticized the idea of this Ukrainian Jew turning out Italian food in New York. She wasn't a chef; she was a cook, and the only reason she was that was because her husband, a southern Italian immigrant who had converted to marry her, was killed at age twenty-two in a streetcar accident. For a young widow there was nothing glamorous about turning out ravioli at work and kreplach at home; it was survival for her and her two little children. She died, having wed three more times, when I was twelve years old; I remember her as a slight, wiry woman who, to the end of her long life, would take her tea in a glass with a cube of sugar held between her teeth. She would have laughed heartily at the idea of her great-granddaughter making a living, in part, by celebrating restaurant cooks in the pages of a glossy magazine.

But that is what happened: I was asked to cover celebrity chefs for the magazine where I work. As I began to navigate their world, I was eating more and richer food than I probably ever have. There were lunches with chefs' publicists, restaurant opening parties, celebrity chef charity events, three- and four-day food festivals, each one a carnival of one-upmanship with sauté pans or tiny blowtorches.

Inconveniently, this occurred in my mid-thirties, as I evolved from being able to eat anything with little consequence to noticing a direct correlation between my morning bagel and a new uncooperativeness from the top button of my jeans. Clearly this would not be allowed to continue, I thought. But I was unwilling to go on a diet. Eating was a big thing for me.

In the course of a few weeks I ate caramelized quail and apple confit at the open-kitchen counter of French chef Joël

Robuchon's L'Atelier at a press lunch in the middle of what would otherwise have been (like the day before and the day after) a sandwich-at-my-desk afternoon; I tasted Rick Moonen's Everything-crusted Tuna (basically all the toppings of an "everything" bagel seared onto a gorgeous ruby piece of fish) at a farewell party for the old Oceana before it closed its town house and moved to the other side of the city; I then met two food-magazine pals at the new, relocated Oceana, and was reminded that when you're in the company of a recognizable and beloved food editor, the chef will send over nearly everything on the menu. Much of that lunch is a blur.

Then the cycle would start again: I'd meet a PR rep for lunch at a client's restaurant, and regardless of how lightly I'd ordered, extra dishes from the kitchen would appear. I'd ask for plain grilled chicken and, in addition, out would come bites of pâté on brioche toast, salads dotted with sweetbreads, a dessert plate composed of six variations on chocolate and cream. Basic politeness (plus a voice in my head—it may have been my great-grandmother's—telling me not to waste food) demanded I taste everything. Sometimes it was more than a taste. By the time you get to that sixth variation of chocolate, you might need to go back and remind yourself about the first. Then the second . . .

Further compounding the problem was the fact that my entry into the food world coincided with what could be called the Bacon Age: a culinary era that, transcending haute and low cuisine, celebrated all things streaky, fatty, smoked, and salty. Bacon appeared in seemingly every dish, from dorade to doughnuts, and made oblivious converts of vegetarians. (Look away if you must, but if that restaurant's green beans taste so much better than the ones you cook at home, credit a pig—not just the chef.) I had never been much of a meat person, but I happily tried what was put in front of me and found some of it delicious, even as I felt that this wasn't really how I was meant to be eating.

Meanwhile, none of this professional exploration took into account the dining I was doing on my own time, like taking my son for the pizza *pane frattau* at Mario Batali's Otto. That's the pizza topped by a fried egg. At the age of six the boy got a "why didn't I think of this" look on his face when he encountered the magical mash-up of two favorite comfort foods. So, clearly I would not be cutting those experiences out of my life.

How were other people, particularly those in the field, handling the problem of too much food, too much temptation, leading to too much person? I was meeting a lot of chefs, and it was impossible not to notice two things: First, they loved food and appeared not to be particularly dainty eaters. Second, they weren't all fat. Yes, some brilliant chefs were pretty big—but they were no longer the norm. In fact, the opposite was true: I met many, many slender and fit chefs. You've seen those folks as well, and you may have wondered how they managed it. I wondered too. Perhaps if I knew what slim chefs did, I could learn to enjoy more and worry less. I had let bagels go, at least on weekdays, because it didn't seem a great sacrifice. But what if, in an attempt to stay in my skinny jeans, I inadvertently eliminated the excitement and flavor from my meals? Or gave up foods that I love? How could I strike the proper balance between pleasure and caution?

The idea for this book started for me with a very simple question: How do chefs eat? We know a lot about how they cook: We can watch them on television, dine in their restaurants, and even, if we're inclined, attempt to re-create their most elaborate dishes at home. But how do people who have dedicated most of their waking hours to food actually feed themselves? Surely not each night with the twelve-course tasting menus they create. Nor did it seem likely to me that they were leaving their own haute cuisine kitchens only to run home and microwave Lean Cuisine.

Since I had access to great chefs, I began talking with them, asking how they ate on the job, or at home with their kids, or when they went out to let someone else do the cooking. I asked about their workouts, and which, if any, foods they cut down on, and which ones they enjoyed most often when they wanted to drop a few pounds. I asked how they ate before the marathon of tasting that comes with judging a TV food competition or testing variations on a dish for one of their own restaurants. I asked what they ate when no one else was looking.

It was Rick Moonen who reminded me that "chefs eat like shit" a lot of the time. (His salty words, though many of his colleagues echoed the idea.) So why ask chefs how to eat or stay in shape? There are nutritionists and dieticians and doctors of several stripes who have dedicated their working lives to these topics. (Not to mention all the skinny actresses and models who will tell you how they do it, though one suspects it doesn't involve many interesting meals—or, for that matter, many meals at all.) But their advice often seems divorced from real life. Notes chef Michael Psilakis, who lost over eighty pounds on a plan of his own design, "Doctors are looking at the problem from a very scientific perspective: This is what you should eat. But what if you *want* to eat something else? There has to be another way." By making chefs the experts, that other way of eating would value flavor above all.

Moonen offers what I think is as good an answer as any to the question of, *Why ask chefs*: "Chefs are fun, and they drink, and people don't want to give that up. There's a happiness factor."

Yes! But here's a more prosaic reason: Chefs work long hours, eat irregularly, and are frequently tempted by an abundance of rich foods. If *they* can maintain a healthy weight, or even lose weight, surely the rest of us can. A chef's life is a magnifying mirror reflection of many of our own. Who among us isn't working hard, fitting in meals, and often tempted by the abundance of food—both good and bad—that is everywhere? But the people who make their living with butter or duck confit or chocolate and still look amazing—they must know some secrets. I wanted in on those secrets. Chefs are intentional about food. What they choose to cook has meaning and is always considered. The chefs in this book have extended that thoughtfulness not just to cooking, but to eating. Which is not to say that how they eat is how they serve us: It was a relief to learn that when Thomas Keller—renowned for creating menus that are as precise as they are lavish—wants a snack, he reaches for a banana or a handful of walnuts; nothing that requires a mandoline or microplane.

For this project, I sought out not necessarily the skinniest chefs—though many are very slender. Instead, I wanted those who are fit, those who make being healthy a priority, and those who have struggled with extra pounds and found solutions that work for them. Inside are stories from chefs who have lost fifteen, twenty-five, forty, eighty, and a hundred pounds.

What I didn't want (and this meant passing over some great new talent) were very young chefs who are slim by virtue of metabolism alone. Everyone here is thirty-something or older. Chefs with long careers and established reputations also happen to be the ones who are in the stage of life when it becomes hard to maintain your current weight, and harder still to lose. I wanted Jedi masters of the kitchen, who have lived and worked around food for decades and come to an understanding with it.

I went to people like Nancy Silverton, of Los Angeles's legendary La Brea Bakery and Osteria Mozza, who cuts a very trim figure despite building her reputation first on bread and then on cheese. And to Chicago's Rick Bayless, who, at fifty-eight, again weighed what he did at eighteen. And to Cat Cora of *Iron Chef*, who is raising four boys while overseeing restaurants and somehow finds time to exercise daily. I also sought input from two restaurateurs with unique perspectives on working around food, as well as a few notable cookbook authors who face similar challenges on the job. I'm grateful that everyone participated with such enthusiasm, sharing personal stories, their weaknesses, their clever tricks, their scrumptious recipes, and, most of all, their valuable time.

The result of their generosity and my efforts is here, presented as ninety-two lessons in living and eating. They include practical tips for, among other things, dining out wisely; cooking at home with the insight (but not the hard-to-replicate professional skills) of a trained chef; keeping dessert and other treats in your life; and making the balance between eating well and living well as simple as possible.

Several tips I found rather surprising: Eric Ripert, of the four-star seafood temple Le Bernardin, will sometimes come home and cook chicken in the toaster oven, a trick he learned from his (nonchef) wife. Chefs known for steak had secret vegetarian lives. Quite a few ate chocolate daily—that was definitely something I wanted to do too.

I took all their ideas seriously, trying to fit these lessons into my own life. It wasn't hard. When, for instance, Michelle Bernstein in Miami would talk about craving a lot of fruit and salads and finishing lunch with a biscotti and espresso, I found I could go for that too. Some of the advice is, admittedly, contradictory: A few of the chefs try to limit their eating to only sit-down meals, while others feel better if they graze throughout the day. I tried both methods—though naturally not in the same day. I invite you to do the same, and find out which chefs' approaches suit you best.

After speaking with more than three dozen chefs, how I ate evolved. I tried new foods and new techniques at home. I ate out with more insight, and even found renewed inspiration when I tied up my running shoes. I remain enchanted by a beautiful meal at a great restaurant, and I have no delusion that I'll ever cook like a professional chef. But armed with their knowledge, I've learned how to eat like a smart chef, and I'm eager to share their wisdom with you.

SMART CHEFS STAY SLIM

Nate Appleman, the culinary manager at Chipotle, won the James Beard Foundation's Rising Star Chef and *Food & Wine*'s Best New Chef in 2009. He is a co-author of *A16 Food + Wine*.

Donatella Arpaia is owner of Donatella in New York, author of *Donatella Cooks,* and a judge on *The Next Iron Chef*.

Joe Bastianich is co-owner of twenty-two restaurants, including Babbo and Del Posto, three wineries, and the New York food emporium Eataly. He is the author of *Grandi Vini* and a judge on *MasterChef*.

Rick Bayless, chef-owner of the Frontera restaurant group in Chicago, has earned six James Beard honors, including Humanitarian of the Year, 1998. The first winner of *Top Chef Masters*, he has written many books and hosts *Mexico—One Plate at a Time* on PBS.

Michelle Bernstein, chef-owner of Michy's, Sra. Martinez and Crumb on Parchment bakery in Miami, was 2007's James Beard Best Chef: South.

Mark Bittman, author of *Food Matters: A Guide to Conscious Eating*, *How to Cook Everything* (winner of the IACP Julia Child award), and many other books, is a columnist for the *New York Times*.

Tom Colicchio, chef-owner of Craft restaurants and Colicchio & Sons, is head judge of *Top Chef*, 2010 James Beard Outstanding Chef, and author of three books, including *Think Like a Chef*.

Cat Cora is an owner of Kouzzina in Orlando, CCQ in Costa Mesa, and Cat Cora's Kitchen at SFO; the author of three books; and an original *Iron Chef America* star.

Gregory Gourdet is chef de cuisine at Departure Restaurant + Lounge in Portland, Oregon. He was a *Food & Wine* People's Best New Chef nominee in 2011.

Laurent Gras was a *Food & Wine* Best New Chef in 2002, and executive chef and partner at Chicago's L20 when it earned three Michelin stars in 2010.

Alexandra Guarnaschelli is executive chef at Butter and the Darby in New York, a judge on *Chopped*, and the host of *The Cooking Loft* and *Alex's Day Off*.

Karen Hatfield and **Quinn Hatfield** are pastry chef and chef, respectively, of Hatfield's in Los Angeles, which they own, along with Sycamore Kitchen. In 2010 Hatfield's was named one of *Bon Appetit*'s 10 Best New Restaurants.

Thomas Keller is the first American chef to hold three Michelin stars at two restaurants: Per Se in New York City, and French Laundry in Yountville, California, which twice topped *Restaurant* magazine's ranking of the Top 50 Restaurants of the World. He is also chef-owner of Bouchon, Bouchon Bakery and ad hoc, and a co-author of several cookbooks.

Matt Lee and **Ted Lee** won the James Beard 2007 Cookbook of the Year award for *The Lee Bros. Southern Cookbook*.

Susur Lee is chef-owner of Lee in Toronto and executive consulting chef of Zentan in Washington, D.C. He is author of *Susur: A Culinary Life*.

Lachlan Mackinnon-Patterson, chef-owner of Frasca Food and Wine in Boulder, Colorado, was a 2005 *Food & Wine* Best New Chef and 2008 James Beard Best Chef: Southwest.

Mark McEwan is chef-owner of Fabbrica, ONE, North 44, and Bymark in Toronto, and the head judge of *Top Chef Canada*.

Rick Moonen, chef-owner of rm seafood in Las Vegas, and author of *Fish Without a Doubt*, was a finalist on *Top Chef Masters*.

Masaharu Morimoto, executive chef of Morimoto restaurants in New York, Philadelphia, Boca Raton, Napa, and Waikiki, is a star of both the Japanese and U.S. editions of *Iron Chef*.

Marc Murphy, executive chef-owner of Benchmarc restaurants, including Landmarc and Ditch Plains in New York, is a judge on *Chopped*.

Melissa Perello is chef-owner of Frances in San Francisco, which earned a Michelin star and was one of *Bon Appetit*'s 10 Best Restaurants in America, 2010.

Naomi Pomeroy, chef-owner of Beast in Portland, Oregon, was a 2009 *Food & Wine* Best New Chef and 2010 finalist for the James Beard Best Chef: Pacific Northwest.

Michael Psilakis is chef-owner of Kefi, Fish Tag, and MP Taverna in New York. *Bon Appetit's* 2008 Chef of the Year, he is author of *How to Roast a Lamb*.

Wolfgang Puck is chef-owner of Spago, which received two Michelin stars, and other restaurants in the United States, Tokyo, Singapore, London, and Toronto, and author of several cookbooks.

Andrea Reusing, chef-owner of Lantern in Chapel Hill, North Carolina, won the 2011 James Beard Award for Best Chef: Southeast. She is the author of *Cooking in the Moment*.

Eric Ripert is chef and co-owner of Le Bernardin, creative director of 10 Arts in Philadelphia, and of Westend Bistro in Washington, D.C. He is the recipient of France's Légion d'Honneur.

Marcus Samuelsson is chef-owner of Red Rooster Harlem and cofounder of the Marcus Samuelsson Group. He received the 2003 James Beard Award for Best Chef: New York City, and won *Top Chef Masters*.

Nancy Silverton, head baker and co-owner of La Brea Bakery, and chef and co-owner of Pizzeria Mozza and Osteria Mozza, won the 1991 James Beard Award for Outstanding Pastry Chef. She is the author of *The Mozza Cookbook* and others.

Art Smith, executive chef and co-owner of Table Fifty-Two in Chicago, Art and Soul in Washington, D.C., Southern Art and Bourbon Bar in Atlanta, and executive chef of Joanne in New York City, received the 2007 James Beard Award for Humanitarian of the Year.

Alessandro Stratta, former executive chef and owner of Alex at Wynn Las Vegas, which earned two Michelin stars, received the 1998 James Beard Award for Best Chef: Southwest. He is a consulting chef for Bigoli in New York City.

Michael Symon is chef-owner of Lola, Lolita, and B Spot in Cleveland, and Michael Symon's Roast in Detroit. The co-author of *Michael Symon's Live to Cook*, he won the 2009 James Beard Award for Best Chef: Great Lakes.

Jacques Torres, owner of Jacques Torres Chocolates, won the 1994 James Beard Award for Outstanding Pastry Chef while at Le Cirque. He is the author of *Dessert Circus* and other books.

Sue Torres is chef-owner of Sueños and consulting executive chef of Rusty Knot, both in New York. She has been a judge on *Chopped* and *Iron Chef America*.

Ming Tsai is chef-owner of Blue Ginger in Wellesley, Massachusetts, and host and executive producer of PBS's *Simply Ming*. He received the 2002 James Beard Award for Best Chef: Northeast.

David Waltuck was the chef and co-owner of Chanterelle in New York City, winner of the James Beard Award for Outstanding Restaurant. He is executive chef for Ark Restaurants.

Simpson Wong is chef-owner of Wong and Café Asean, and formerly of Jefferson, all in New York City.

Sang Yoon is chef-owner of Lukshon in Culver City and Father's Office in Santa Monica and Los Angeles; his Office Burger was voted best burger in the country in two popular polls.

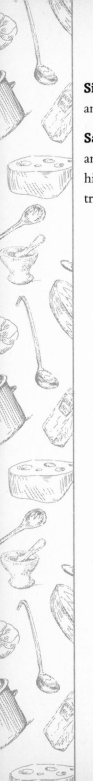

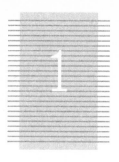

EAT WHAT
YOU LOVE

I'M GOING TO put the best thing I heard in all my interviews right out front: *Eat the food you love.*

One of the great pleasures in talking to chefs is hearing these pros go all swoony over the dishes, or the simple ingredients, that they adore. Ming Tsai thinks a late-night bowl of ramen is "freakin' delicious." When she lived in Paris as a young chef, Alex Guarnaschelli used to keep a quart of cream in her refrigerator and take a sip from it every so often, just because "I love the taste of French cream," she tells me. Michelle Bernstein: "My mother's carrot cake—one of the best things I've had in my life." Marc Murphy: "Steak, sweetbreads, a little foie gras terrine . . ."

How can any of these foods stay in a person's life and not cause those who partake to pack on the pounds? For one, there is a big difference between eating *only* what you love and eating whatever you like. Eating what you love means limiting yourself to only the foods you really, truly enjoy and not wasting time (or calories or fat grams or net carbs or whatever it makes you feel good to count) eating what you do not absolutely adore. Eating this way relies on the notion that if you get exactly what you want, you don't need a lot of it. It is not as if Guarnaschelli was downing a glass of cream a day; just a sip was enough. More is not necessarily better.

Because they include the foods they love, chefs' diets, even when restrained, remain a source of pleasure. An eating plan that is filled with food you love is one that's pretty easy to stick to. Here, a few more philosophies to bring to the table.

Lesson 1: Smart chefs surround themselves with real food they love

"People don't realize you can eat a lot of good food—but you can't eat garbage food," says Michael Psilakis, chef at the first Greek restaurant in America to earn a Michelin star. He achieved a major slim-down—the kind that reality shows with before-and-after photos are built on—by eating many of the things he loves. (He shares the details in Chapter 14.) So what does he mean by good food? For one, dishes made from high-quality, real ingredients that are minimally processed. But no less important: food that tastes good to him.

Rick Bayless, America's dean of Mexican cuisine, shares that perspective: "My life is all about good food," says Bayless, a fourth-generation restaurateur and chef for more than thirty years. Today Bayless is as slender as he was as a young man in Oklahoma City. One reason? "When you eat good food, it satisfies you and you don't have to be gluttonous about it. I'd rather have one bite of a great dish than fifty bites of a mediocre dish," he says.

If that seems an obvious point—who wouldn't rather have great food than mediocre?—consider how often we settle for less than spectacular. For instance, what did you have for lunch yesterday? (Me: a spongy chicken banh mi from the sandwich shop next to my office; won't get that again.) Think of all the times when you eat something so-so, because it was more convenient, or cheaper, or faster.

The solution is to replace the so-so with the great. But for you to do that, great food needs to be available. That means keeping the great food you love on hand in your kitchen, choosing restaurants that serve it, and even sometimes packing your own lunch in order to avoid the sad food often consumed at a desk. This took me ages to learn and I really fought it: Can a person who can barely decide what to have for breakfast really be expected to plan lunch at the same time?

It helps to think of the home kitchen a bit like a restaurant kitchen, not in terms of preparing fancy meals, but in terms of stocking the basics of your menu. "What I want to eat is the stuff that is going to keep me the size I am," says Bayless. Me too. So that means that this week I'm probably going to eat at least one meal that includes salmon, another with some kind of canned bean—I'm terrible at remembering to soak dried beans ahead of time—a few that include some salad or spinach, and I'm going to want some Greek yogurt most mornings and I'll be grumpy if there isn't ripe fruit to go with it. In the extremely exclusive restaurant that is my apartment dining room, these are the usuals, and I need to keep a constant supply of the components that make up these meals (if yogurt and a banana qualifies as a meal). You know how you feel when you go to an actual restaurant and they have eighty-sixed your favorite dish? Don't do that to yourself.

Bayless has made it easy: When he's home in Chicago he eats from his own menus at Topolobampo or Frontera Grill or

XOCO twice a day. "It's how I keep track of what it's like to be a guest," he explains. But if he's away, and good food isn't readily available, Bayless won't nosh on whatever junk is around. "My family laughs at me about this, but I'll skip a meal if I don't think there's anything good enough to eat."

Don't suppose that Bayless is skipping a lot of meals. On the contrary, he makes a point of affording himself great eating opportunities, whether he's going out, or on the job at the restaurant, or taping his PBS show. "I feel so blessed, because I'm around really good food all the time. People who don't work around food are always thinking that because I'm surrounded by good food that I'm just going to gobble it, I'm going to eat it all of the time, because who can resist? But the *more* you're around good food and appreciate it, the *less* you have to have to be satisfied."

I got a crash course in implementing this philosophy at the place where I first meet Bayless—the South Beach Wine & Food Festival, a four-day charity event in Miami with scads of celebrity and local chefs outdoing one another. This isn't an environment that lends itself to moderation. He is serving pulled-pork tacos, a nod to his parents' barbecue restaurant and his own haute Mexican cuisine. They are one of several dozen barbecue dishes on offer at the festival's famous "BubbleQ," a barbecue with champagne. His taco is a perfect few bites. But also here are offerings from Bobby Flay and Jonathan Waxman and Elizabeth Karmel and Todd English, and the list goes on. Do I need to try all the barbecue? Of course not. I congratulate myself on showing restraint. Later, at another tasting party, I completely blow it at the dessert table. What can I say? It's a process. Did I really *love* all those desserts I sampled? No, not really.

Lesson learned: If something doesn't offer a lot of pleasure, I should not be eating it. Have I ever craved the taste of a protein bar? No, never. Have I ever wolfed down a greasy bag of movie popcorn and thought, "That was *delicious*—even better than the film"? No, not once. (Okay, possibly once, during the last hour of the interminable Tom Cruise sci-fi fake-out *Vanilla Sky*. But other than that, no.) Have I ever finished a boring restaurant meal because I was paying for it or, for that matter, because I *wasn't* paying for it? Cut out food about which you are unenthusiastic, and you'll save countless wasted calories.

Lesson 2: They never feel guilty about eating what they love

Le Bernardin's Eric Ripert tells me is he asked in interviews, "What is your guilty pleasure?" He's flummoxed each time. "To me it is inconceivable to have guilt about eating," says the Antibes-born chef. "I was educated from a young age to eat good food—good-quality ingredients, and in moderation. Feeling guilty about eating is an American idea. When you eat and you feel guilt, it's not edifying; you're just putting things in your stomach. Maybe that is why people are overweight?" he ventures.

If there are no "guilty pleasures," does it then follow that there are no foods that you can never eat? Chefs would say there's nothing that you should *never* eat. Deciding to ban a particular food, or group of foods, is not an easy option for chefs, who prefer to have the full spectrum of flavors and textures available to them. Furthermore, says Craft's Tom Colicchio, "Diets don't work when you tell people they can't have something. You can eat anything; it's about eating less. I'm eating fewer 'white things' but haven't cut them out." (White things = white bread, white sugar, white potatoes.)

Rather than put foods on the banned list, chefs enjoy them less frequently. In that previous sentence you may feel that the key phrase is "less frequently." Fair enough. I would argue that equally significant is "enjoy them." Once in a while, enjoy your favorites—really enjoy them, no guilt. A sampling of chefs and their once-in-a-while treats:

Blue Ginger's Ming Tsai says, "I can go without sweets," but he won't give up fried foods. "I mean, come on—onion rings? French fries? Potato chips?"

"Sweets and bread are my downfall," says Wolfgang Puck of Spago in Beverly Hills. "My favorite thing is coffee macarons. I tell our pastry chef, 'Why don't you make coffee macarons, for a cookie plate?' Then she makes them, and I eat them. Then I tell her, 'Why did you make coffee macarons? You know I eat them,'" he says, laughing.

"They used to call me the queen of foie gras, because I ordered more foie and used more foie than anybody in Miami," says Sra. Martinez chef-owner Michelle Bernstein. "I would make it for someone, taste a little bit. Make some, taste some more. I still serve it sometimes, but now I'm eating it maybe once a year." Indeed, she lived up to her old title for a food festival event, making hundreds of small portions of foie gras mousse with kumquat gelée, duck rillettes, and chicharon salad. That's more like a once-in-a-decade concoction.

In addition to not denying themselves completely, smart chefs come up with coping rules so that they can happily enjoy their favorite foods mindfully, with some boundaries. Bread was often cited as a must-have, but with some caveats.

"If I eat bread at home, it's special bread that someone made," says Andrea Reusing of Chapel Hill's Lantern restaurant. "My brothers and I always made fun of my mom when we wanted white bread and she'd say, 'Empty calories! It's just empty calories!' But that's the right approach: to never eat empty calories. Eating things that are nutritionally dense is good."

Once in a while Rick Moonen, in Las Vegas, likes to treat himself to an In-N-Out burger, but says he can do without the bread. He orders the not-on-the-menu "protein wrap," which is a burger with all the fixings tucked into iceberg lettuce leaves instead of a bun. "You have to know to ask for it," he tells me furtively. "Wink-wink, say no more."

Nancy Silverton made her name in the Los Angeles food scene with the La Brea Bakery; there's no way she's giving up bread. "I eat some bread every day. I don't know when [low-carb diets] became such an obsession, but it was a few years after we opened the bakery," recalls Silverton. "We thought we would feel some backlash. But what we found was that it really didn't affect us—it almost helped us. Rather than people eliminating all carbohydrates from their diet, I think it made them choose more carefully. People requested more whole-grain than just white-flour bread. Rather than eating an inferior bread daily, they would eat it less frequently, but choose quality and better taste."

Lesson 3: They are picky eaters

Donatella Arpaia is adamant about never finishing a blah dish—even if it is one she ordered herself. "If I don't like something, or it is not exactly what I want, I won't eat it," says Arpaia, owner of Donatella in New York, as well as a cooking school grad who could have been a contender in the kitchen. "I just stop. I don't care. I got over my thing about wasting food and leaving your plate half-full."

I'm not advocating for wastefulness—few things offend me

more, save for competitive eating contests. (Is *that* the way to honor our country on the Fourth of July? I think not.) But once the food reaches your plate, it does seem wise to eat only what is appealing and leave behind anything not that exciting. Don't eat it out of obligation, or just because it's there.

This was a practice Arpaia figured out over time. "Because I'm a woman, and I was younger than most people in this industry when I started, everyone was constantly dissecting my body. Every day I got a comment: 'You look fat.' 'You look skinny.' 'You look *much* better now.' You kidding me? And it was always fat old men saying this."

She learned to tune out the comments, but still had her own reasons for wanting to watch how she eats. "I like clothes. How am I going to stay thin, but do what I do? I had to create rules for myself. When I was younger I would clean my plate, two portions full." Or she would catch herself eating a dessert that didn't really knock her socks off, just because it had been placed before her. "Now," says Arpaia, "if I'm going to have chocolate, it's going to be Payard, the best chocolate, and I'm going to enjoy it and eat a small portion of it instead of something inferior, like sugar-free cookies."

It is a strong argument for a little snobbism, I think. Once I started thinking of myself as the kind of person who eats only the best chocolate, the great wall of candy bars at the grocery checkout became all but invisible to me. The vending machine just steps away from my office door? I no longer think of it as containing anything edible; it's more like an art installation celebrating things I used to eat at four p.m., when I was desperate for sugar and salt.

Picky eating isn't just for grown-ups. Raising your kid as a (polite, well-mannered) food snob is fun too. I knew that I didn't want my son to eat only chicken fingers and buttered noodles from children's menus, and so made an effort to introduce him to great food early. But just as important as getting him hooked on real food was teaching him what *not* to eat. At a young age, he was let in on a grown-up secret: "They need the clown and the toys in the meals because the food is so terrible," I told him, "and why would you want to eat terrible food?" Which doesn't mean he never gets French fries, just infrequently, and never from a clown. It's a lot easier to learn good habits early than to have to unlearn them later.

Lesson 4: They know exactly what they want to eat

You might be able to say, in general, which foods you love. But what do you feel like eating right now? Chefs think about food *a lot*. It doesn't mean they necessarily always eat what they are thinking about, but we should all be so in tune with our own desires. Says New York chef Alex Guarnaschelli, "You can't not honor the love and temptation you feel toward food and stay true to yourself. You might be thinner, but you lose something." Guarnaschelli was cautious when I approached her to find out how she eats. Although she achieved a sixty-pound post-baby weight loss, she still considers herself very much a work in progress. "It's something I'm learning: the idea of staying true to what you want to eat and cook."

When you deny yourself what you're craving in favor of something you believe you're supposed to eat, you're left wanting. Better to get what you *really* want, and eat only that. Acclaimed pastry chef and chocolatier Jacques Torres knows what to eat to lose weight—he dropped thirty pounds while remaining on full-time Willy Wonka duty. What he also knows is that if what you really want some evening is a baguette and a round of vacherin, there is very little point in making yourself steamed fish and vegetables. Somehow, after your virtuous dinner, you will find a way to get bread and cheese, even if it requires digging like a gopher to the back wall of your refrigerator, only to locate the lowly substitute of a smear of cream cheese on the rump end of pumpernickel. (Yes, it is possible this is a scenario drawn from my own life; who needs to know?) So sometimes he will say to his wife, Hasty, a chocolatier with her own shop, "How about we have cheese for dinner?"

Can he do this every night? No, of course not. It would be irresponsible to let you believe you can eat cheese for dinner nightly and not put on weight. But by letting himself *occasionally* indulge in a bread, wine, and cheese dinner that looks like a Seurat picnic, he avoids looking like a Botero.

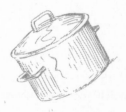

Rick Bayless's Grilled Chicken Salad with Rustic Guacamole

This simple dish uses chilies, lime, and cilantro to transcend the dieter's staple of salad and chicken. And it's dead easy: You make a batch of the sauce, then use a third of it to marinate the chicken, a third of it to season the guacamole, and the final third to dress the salad. Remarkably, this repeated usage doesn't taste like sameness, but like different notes in close harmony. While I am generally a proponent of forging ahead with a recipe even when you don't have every last ingredient, I urge you not to leave off the sprinkling of aged cheese—those sorts of small additions add flavor and satisfaction.

serves 4

FOR THE DRESSING:

½ cup vegetable or olive oil, plus a little more for
   the onion
4 garlic cloves, peeled and cut in half lengthwise
Fresh hot green chilies to taste (Rick likes 2 serranos or 1 large jalapeño), stemmed and halved
½ cup fresh lime juice
¾ cup (loosely packed) roughly chopped cilantro
¼ teaspoon ground black pepper
Salt to taste

FOR THE SALAD:

4 medium (about 1¼ pounds total) boneless, skin-
   less chicken breast halves
1 medium white onion, cut into ½-inch slices
2 ripe avocados

**Romaine hearts, sliced crosswise at ½-inch thick
(about 8 cups)
About ⅓ cup grated Mexican *queso añejo* (or
pecorino Romano or Parmesan)**

1. Heat the oil in a small skillet over medium heat. Add the garlic and chilies, and cook, stirring frequently, until the garlic is soft and lightly browned, about 1 to 2 minutes. Place the oil, garlic, and chilies into a blender or food processor. Add the lime juice, cilantro, and 1 scant teaspoon salt and ¼ teaspoon black pepper. Process until smooth. Pour ⅓ of the garlic mixture over the chicken breasts, spreading it evenly over all sides.

2. Heat a gas grill or grill pan over medium to medium-high (or start a charcoal fire and let it burn until the coals are medium-hot and covered with white ash). Lightly brush or spray the onion slices with oil; sprinkle both sides with salt. Lay the chicken and onion on the grill or grill pan. Cook until the chicken is just cooked through and the onion is well browned, 3 to 4 minutes on each side.

3. Chop the onion into small pieces and place into a small bowl. Pit and peel the avocados, scooping the flesh, and add to the bowl with the onion. Add another ⅓ of the garlic mixture, then coarsely mash everything together with an old-fashioned potato masher, large fork, or back of spoon. Taste and season with salt, usually about ½ teaspoon.

4. Place the sliced romaine into a large bowl. Drizzle on the remaining ⅓ of the garlic mixture and toss to combine. Divide between 4 dinner plates. Scoop a portion of the guacamole into the center of each plate. Cut each breast into cubes and arrange over the guacamole. Sprinkle each plate with the grated cheese. Serve.

Adapted from *Mexican Everyday* by Rick Bayless with Deann Groen Bayless. W. W. Norton and Company, 2005.

———

Wolfgang Puck's Provençal Salmon with Tomato-basil Sauce

The sauce can be made a day ahead, so on a weeknight all you will have to do is broil the fish. A nonreactive bowl is one made from glass or stainless steel—not plastic, copper, or most other metals, which can react to the acid in foods like lemon or tomatoes. One more thing: Don't freeze; fresh tomatoes don't do well after being frozen and thawed.

serves 4

FOR THE SAUCE:

- 3 large ripe tomatoes, peeled, seeded, and finely chopped
- 2 small shallots, minced
- ½ cup chopped fresh organic basil leaves
- ½ teaspoon lemon zest, finely grated, or more to taste
- ⅓ cup extra-virgin olive oil
- 4 teaspoons sherry wine vinegar
- 2 teaspoons minced fresh chives
- 2 teaspoons minced fresh tarragon
- Salt and freshly ground pepper to taste
- Cayenne pepper to taste

FOR THE SALMON:

**4 salmon fillets, about 6 ounces each, preferably
  wild-caught from Alaska**
Extra-virgin olive oil
Salt and freshly ground pepper to taste
6 small sprigs fresh organic basil for garnish

1. Make the sauce several hours in advance or the night before. In a nonreactive mixing bowl stir together the tomatoes, shallots, basil, lemon zest, olive oil, vinegar, chives, and tarragon. Season to taste with salt, pepper, and a little cayenne. Cover the bowl and leave at room temperature to marinate for several hours or overnight in the refrigerator to allow the flavors to meld.

2. About ½ hour before serving time, preheat the oven to 400°F. Cover a baking sheet with foil and lightly oil the foil. Brush the salmon fillets with olive oil, season them with salt and pepper, and arrange them on a baking sheet. Cook until the top is very lightly browned and the flesh is still slightly pink in the center, 7 to 8 minutes, depending on thickness of the fish. Meanwhile, taste the sauce and, if necessary, adjust the seasonings to taste.

3. Spoon a generous amount of the sauce onto the middle of each of 6 heated serving plates. Place the salmon fillets on top of the sauce. Top each fillet with a basil sprig. Serve immediately, passing any remaining sauce separately.

Adapted from *Wolfgang Puck Makes It Easy* by Wolfgang Puck.
Rutledge Hill Press, 2004.

BEHIND THE LESSONS:

Alexandra Guarnaschelli's
Twitter Feed

One of my favorite digital-age pastimes is following chefs on Twitter.com. Fans use it to connect with celebrities, and I admit that I've used it to publically express my thanks for a recipe that worked well or to ask a cooking question and—voilà!—get an answer. By just observing throughout any given day, you can get 140-character glimpses into the food they are preparing, serving, eating, or daydreaming about.

In my opinion, the lyric poet of this extremely modern form is Alex Guarnaschelli, the executive chef of Butter restaurant and the Darby, a supper club, both in New York City. Alex is the daughter of a professor/therapist father (who used to make her meatballs) and a mother who is the noted editor of, among many, many other cookbooks, the 1997 edition of *The Joy of Cooking*, which, incidentally, was the first engagement gift I received. Perhaps that combination of genes somehow contributed to her perceptive and sensual writing about food, even on this new, strange, small scale. Here, a few of her musings:

> **27 Feb @guarnaschelli**—Cannot stop thinking about a slice of warm, freshly baked onion bread with cream cheese (that melts ever so slightly), smoked salmon, lemon.

> **5 April @guarnaschelli**—Have you ever dunked a french fry in ketchup and felt a small sizzle as the hot fry meets the super cold ketchup?

23 April @guarnaschelli—Roasted asparagus with shaved Parmesan, black pepper, lemon, and a poached egg. Egg oozes so elegantly.

10 May @guarnaschelli—Seriously browned pork sausage links w parsley, garlic, onions. Fried egg on top, toasted brioche w cinnamon, salted butter. Criminally good.

26 June @guarnaschelli—Roasted some apricots and raspberries and topped with a scoop of olive oil ice cream. Unreal.

"I have a love affair with food, for sure," Alex tells me. "What I write on Twitter is true. People say, 'This isn't you.' How could it *not* be me? At four a.m. I'm eating fried chicken in the fridge—that's not me? Come on."

What moves her to write a quick culinary mash note? "Sometimes it's something I eat; sometimes it's something I cook for someone else; sometimes it's something I see that makes me want it," says Alex. When I asked, she wouldn't say which of her tweets were daydreams, and which documented what was actually on her plate. "I live in a neighborhood where there are a lot of different foods and I'll walk by a place and say, 'Ooh, I forgot about you!' Food to me can be like old boyfriends: Sometimes they're nicer to think about fleetingly."

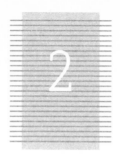

EAT WITH YOUR
EYES OPEN

CHEFS SPEND A lot of time putting food in their mouths without really eating. By which I don't mean that they are spitting out the food. (Ew. Don't do that.) But for pros, there's a difference between "tasting" and "eating." If eating is for pleasure or sustenance, tasting is for work. They are making sure the meat is seasoned and seared properly. They are dipping into sauces and stocks to monitor salt levels. Throughout an evening, as a sauce reduces it becomes saltier, so chefs check, adjust, and check again. What's this new creation the pastry chef is sending out? Bite. Bite. Bite. Before you notice, we're talking real quantities. Cleveland's Michael Symon echoed many of his colleagues when he told me, "Because of what I do for a living, I consume a giant amount of calories—I would say four to six thousand on a heavy day. I gotta taste."

We layfolk don't have that same professional obligation to taste food throughout the day or night. But think of all the other opportunities we have to nosh, graze, or sample and not count it as eating, because it was "just a bite" (or twenty) or eaten standing up (or while driving), or a taste of someone else's meal (or two-thirds of your kid's unfinished sandwich), or any other number of rationalizations that all those extra bites somehow don't make a difference. They do. Often we don't even notice that we're taking them in. I'm not a big calorie counter, because if there's anything that makes eating less fun, it is math. But just becoming aware of everything that hits your mouth—and of *why* you're putting it in there—can be a meaningful change.

Lesson 5: Smart chefs are awake when they eat

"I try very hard to pay attention to what I put in my mouth all day long," says Melissa Perello of Frances in San Francisco. (The name honors her Texas grandmother, who taught Melissa to cook.) Her menu, which changes almost daily, is heavily market-driven, so she isn't doing dishes by rote—she has to taste to create. "Sometimes I get off track, so I have to be careful. Whenever I feel like my weight's getting out of control, I really try to focus on what I'm eating, keep a mental diary. If I know I already ate x, y, and z, I can say, 'I do not need to eat this piece of cake right now.'"

Michelle Bernstein agrees. "It's something that you have to be cognizant of all day long." Before she was a chef, Bernstein studied with Alvin Ailey in New York and aspired to be a professional dancer. The rigors of the two professions are comparable, but that may be where the similarities end. "As soon as I quit and got into cooking, I immediately felt that I started to gain weight. I wanted to look the same, but it didn't work," says Bernstein, who remains lithe and graceful in the kitchen. "If the pastry chef comes up with three new desserts, you have to taste them—but then you have to *remember* that you tasted them. So later when you drink coffee that day, you shouldn't put sugar in your coffee. Or maybe you shouldn't have that cup of coffee if you have to have sugar in it. Or you don't eat bread later. If my husband says, 'Come have a sandwich with me,' I'll have the inside, not the outside. It's something that you have to think about. Some people use their phones to write down what they're eating. I just try to keep a mental note."

During dinner service, she adds, "You can be tasting and feel like you haven't eaten anything and think, 'I need to sit down and eat something.' Meanwhile, you've already ingested eight hundred to a thousand calories in sauces alone, and enough fat for probably a third of the day."

Her solution: Put down the spoon and pick up a vegetable. "Now I'm dipping lettuce or a carrot so my body doesn't trick my mind into thinking I haven't eaten anything." This is good advice—I tend to pick at whatever is handy when I'm cooking dinner, because most nights, by the time I get to the stove I'm already pretty hungry. Switching to some raw vegetables from bread or cheese was easy, and doing so means I've had something nutritious (but not highly caloric) even before the meal. This also works in other fraught situations, like cocktail parties with sliders circulating on trays and a dessert bar. It's easier to lose track of what you've eaten and overindulge at a party with a buffet or passed hors d'oeuvres than when you sit down to a meal. A few raw vegetables can get you through those grazing situations unscathed, or at least help you feel satisfied with only one slider instead of four.

Lesson 6: **They dine with a strategy**

Naturally there are situations, family holiday gatherings for one, that demand more than just chomping on carrot sticks and red pepper strips. Some planning is helpful in those cases. Donatella Arpaia says that in advance of a big food event, she thinks about what and how much she intends to eat. "I make a mental plan when it's Christmas, and my mom has a twenty-course feast with the meatballs and the chicken cutlets. I say, 'Okay, what are my most favorite things? I'm going to eat that, and that, and that.'" And that's all. The rest, she says, "is a feast for the eyes."

You will—hopefully, inevitably—go to parties with phenomenal food that you want to enjoy, and sometimes your better judgment will abandon you and you'll eat too much. It happens. If you're paying attention, you can simply remember to go light the next day. That is just what Rick Moonen was doing when we spoke—trying to balance out the excesses of the previous day. Moonen had been judging an up-and-coming-chefs competition in Napa. "Ten dishes of one pork preparation. Horrible. I wanted to die." He groaned, less about the food itself than the quantity and heft of it all. "Then I went to the French Laundry because I'm in Yountville—I have to bring my girlfriend to the best restaurant in the world."

It's a good bet that he didn't eat anything bad at Thomas Keller's landmark restaurant. Moonen, who knows Keller, says they were treated to an all-out feast. "We got pummeled. I'm done. Done! So today I'm eating raw." There's nothing to suggest that a full-time diet of uncooked food is especially beneficial, despite what raw foodists would have us believe. But an occasional day of fresh fruits and vegetables, and maybe some nuts for protein, is a reasonable way to get back on track after overindulgence.

Lesson 7: **They know you never enjoy those last bites as much as the first**

This seems a good time to hear from Thomas Keller, the culinary bard behind those extraordinary experiences at the French Laundry and its New York City counterpart, Per Se. He really isn't trying to topple guests with too much food. In fact, to his way of thinking, it's best if you stop eating a dish when you still want more of it. "Our whole menu is based on the law of diminishing returns," Keller explains to me. "It's our philosophy about our food: The most compelling portion of a dish is the first three or four bites. With the first bite you're getting into it, by the second you start to realize it, and it is at the third or fourth bites you get the maximum appreciation and pleasure from that dish—you think, 'This is amazing!' and you keep eating it because of that *memory* of it being really extraordinary. But by the time you're done with it, okay, that was really good, but was it as good [at the end] as it was at that second, third or fourth bite? No."

His solution—smaller portions. If you have a big bunch of something that good, the temptation is to just keep eating and eating, trying in vain to recapture the thrill of that early pleasure. To Keller, the perfect time to part ways from a plate of food is when you are still wishing for one more bite, not when you've had so much that you're tired of it. "People will ask, 'Can I have another cornet?'" he says of a signature canapé (salmon tartare and sweet red onion crème fraîche in a tiny cone studded with black sesame seeds). "They'll say, 'The first one was so good, I want another.' No. It's a matter of finishing a dish at the height of that flavor impact."

At his restaurants, when that moment occurs another small

course is right behind—some new experience to captivate the diner. But the philosophy is worth taking home, and applying to those treats that wow you initially, but diminish with the more you have of them. The tenth spoonful of ice cream. The fourteenth twirl of fettuccine Alfredo. The umpteenth tortilla chip with guacamole. None are as great as that first (or second or third or fourth) time. Have less, savor more.

Lesson 8: They consider why they are eating

"I'm a little bit of a nervous eater," confesses Andrea Reusing. "In the kitchen at night I have to find that line between tasting and stress eating because it's busy. Otherwise I find that I've eaten my day's calories in croutons." Reusing has a warm mushroom salad recipe that I followed at home one night. The croutons, which you make fresh from country bread, olive oil, and salt, were addictively crunchy. As I was assembling the rest of the dinner I found myself snacking away on the croutons, trying to see how many I could pick off before the dish would cease to be something that could be described as "a salad with croutons." (Quite a lot, as it turns out.)

Then there is the problem of what I call "batting cleanup," when there's just a little left in a dish so you finish it off. For a week before heading to Miami, I was eating very carefully and working out—the prospect of putting on a swimsuit in the middle of winter will do that. Then, the night before getting on the plane, I was making a spinach and mushroom lasagna for my son and husband to heat up while I was gone. After I'd made enough layers to fill the pan to the top, there were still a few broken lasagna noodles left in the colander. Although I'd had a satisfying dinner two hours earlier, I snatched those noodles up, mopped them through the puddle of béchamel left in the pot, and ate them standing at the stove. Creamy, lush, slightly springy and . . . *totally unnecessary.* The béchamel, I am ashamed to report, needed more salt and pepper. But as the bulk of it was already mortaring the layers of pasta, spinach, cheese, and mushrooms, this cannot be described as effective tasting, as I could not go back and reseason the sauce. It was mindless Hoovering. The moral of the story: Taste the food you're preparing only when the dish still stands to benefit from some adjustments.

The only way Reusing says she is able to thwart those Hoovering episodes "is just being aware." Once she tuned in to how much she was eating, she realized she should just call all those bites at night what they are: dinner. Rather than try to keep her grazing in check, she stopped sitting down to a meal after a shift of checking her sauces and meats—and saw that she wasn't missing anything. So if you find yourself snacking, just remember that you've done it, and don't eat just as much at the dinner table. If you've had a particularly heavy afternoon of noshing, maybe you skip dinner. Who says we need three squares a day, every day?

Marcus Samuelsson tells me he'd been talking over this very idea with his wife, Maya Haile, a fashion model who is from Ethiopia. "My wife says in Africa, 'We eat one big meal a day. We have tea in the morning, maybe with a hint of bread. Maybe a little bit of coffee. A lot of water during the day, then this one big meal that becomes a celebration.' You know, that's not a bad way," says Samuelsson, who was also born in Ethiopia, but raised in Sweden.

It's not that we should necessarily be skipping meals, he adds, just that we should be making a conscious choice to eat out of hunger, not just habit. "Breakfast-lunch-dinner-breakfast-lunch-dinner-breakfast-lunch-dinner is not the way to go," he says, stringing the words together like a train of boxcars stretching to the horizon. "I don't think I've arrived at the answer yet, but I can tell you that's not it. There are a lot of people in the world who don't eat breakfast-lunch-dinner and they're in great shape." We agree that the first step is observing one's habits, then making adjustments. "Your body can get used to anything: If you have a snack at two p.m. every day, you'll get used to a snack at two p.m. every day," says Samuelsson. "If you change that snack from a muffin to an apple, you'll get used to that too. Bodies become very much accustomed."

Case in point: Thomas Keller says he routinely has a morning and an afternoon snack, and that invariably they are one of the following: an apple, a banana, some almonds or walnuts, or crackers with peanut butter. If you get hungry between meals, better to have an arsenal of reliable, nutritious favorites. And keeping a piece of fruit and some nuts close at hand is no more difficult than hitting a vending machine.

Lesson 9: **Smart chefs don't snack mindlessly**

A divide across the Atlantic: Americans are all-day noshers, Europeans not so much. "I was an adult before I learned the word 'snack,'" says Marcus Samuelsson. In Sweden, he says, "Our parents counted on the meal that the kids got in school. You got a fantastic lunch: always a rye bread, water or milk, fish or meat or a vegetarian dish. It could be seared cod with broccoli and mashed potato. The next day split-pea soup, with a grilled piece of ham and mustard." The meals were hearty, and carried the kids through until the evening. "If you can trust the school to provide that for you, then you can eat as a family at a certain time."

We do a lot of habitual eating in this country. Taking a coffee break? Have a doughnut. Going to a movie? Get popcorn. Watching the Super Bowl? Bring on the nachos. Eric Ripert says he never really saw that type of hand-to-mouth viewing until he moved to the States. "In France you don't go to the movie theater and pick on popcorn," says Ripert, who met with me the morning after the Packers beat the Steelers. "I love the Super Bowl party, but in France it doesn't happen like that. You don't stuff yourself with chicken wings. Maybe the younger generation has a tendency to. But as a tradition, no."

Marc Murphy, an American chef who spent time in France with his mother's family, agrees with Ripert: "People who eat too much are just snacking all the time. I like to sit down and have my meal. I don't like to eat on the subway. I don't even like to have a cup of tea while walking—and I drink a lot of tea."

He's got me beat on that—I do like having a take-out cup of tea when I'm walking around the city in winter. I consider it as much a part of my cold-weather gear as mittens or a scarf. In the summer I tote around an iced coffee with milk, no sugar. Perhaps this is a lesson I still need to learn: Snacks are not accessories. But, after talking with Ripert and Murphy, I did try in earnest to ignore the call to eat between meals. When I first tried cutting out snacks, I noticed I wanted to eat more at breakfast or lunch. I suppose I was worried that I might feel hungry afterward. Well, so what if I did get hungry? Food was never more than a short walk away. Besides, feeling a little hungry—not to the point where you're snapping at coworkers, but so that there is an awareness—can be part of the pleasure before eating. It's okay to not snack and thus to not walk around half-full all the time, I discovered. I really didn't miss snacking as long as I made sure to have a little protein in each meal and not falsely fill up on fluffy foods without depth.

The effect of eating this way was to make my meals more memorable—at the end of the day I actually knew what I ate, and I didn't have to consult a food journal to tell you that today I had two eggs and green tea for breakfast, a piece of (slightly underseasoned) leftover spinach and mushroom lasagna for lunch, and salmon croquettes with broccoli rabe and an arugula/avocado salad for dinner, followed by two squares of dark chocolate. Meals stand out in starker relief if they aren't indistinguishable bumps in an all-day food graph.

Lesson 10: They pull back if they are eating on autopilot

Iron Chef star Cat Cora likes to linger over a great meal as much as the next person. But she figures after about twenty minutes, she's finished with the eating aspect. "Sit down to a meal and savor it and eat for twenty minutes," she says. "If you're still eating after that, you're no longer hungry. It's really about other things. Maybe your palate wants more, or you think you've got to finish, or other people are still eating."

Not to take away from the importance of those elements that can cause us to eat more: Good company, conversation, a long meal with a lot of delicious courses—these are essential in life. But if you pay close attention to your hunger, you'll realize that it gets satisfied much sooner than you think. Says Cora: "Sit back, take a breath, and consider. You'll either say, 'Okay, I'm going to take a couple more bites,' or, 'Wow, I'm not hungry. I'm done.'"

She's right, of course. I rarely need all the food in front of me at most meals, but I don't like to be finished eating too soon. I like being at the table, whether talking with friends or reading the paper by myself. So occasionally I give myself something else to do. For lingerers like me, some great foods are a whole artichoke, in-shell pistachios, or a tangerine that needs to be peeled and each piece depithed—foods that take more work to consume.

Sometimes the opposite can be true: You aren't aware of being sated because you are eating too fast. Slowing down did not come naturally to Cora, who found that between her restaurants, TV shows, and expanding family she was often, she says, "gobbling food down because I'd have only ten minutes to eat." When she actually did have time to sit and linger over a great meal, she would wolf it down in the same record time as she did when she was eating on the run. "I'm as guilty as anyone," she admits. "It took me a while to learn to stop and enjoy my food."

To take an extreme example of long-term dining, a meal at Per Se or the French Laundry can take upward of three and a half hours, during which time customers will encounter nine to fifteen (sometimes eighteen!) tiny courses, adding up to about a pound of food. (With the extended menu, each course is smaller so the total stays about the same.) I ask the chef about serving so much over such a long a time.

"Eating a pound of food is a lot!" Thomas Keller acknowledges, with a laugh. It seems less preposterous as he talks me through the meal. "Maybe the lobster is an ounce and a half, and the fish is an ounce. The foie gras you don't want to skimp on, so that course may be two and a half ounces." Also adding to the bottom line: pre-canapés, canapés, salad, more protein courses and two or three desserts, each one no more than a few bites.

He knows this is not the way anyone eats under normal circumstances—going to his restaurants is, as it should be, a rarified experience that is primarily about delighting one's senses. But even here it is possible to take away a lesson in eating wisely. Menus like this come out of the Japanese tradition, *kaiseki*, of "eating small portions over a long period of time," Keller tells me. "It is a health benefit, to eat slowly and take your time." By contrast, he notes that, "if you're really hungry you could inhale a pound of pasta. You've done it. I've done it. Then you go, 'Oh shit, why did I eat so much?' Why? Because your mind and your body didn't have a chance to sync up on how much you ate. Here, you eat over a long period of time and your mind is talking to your stomach, your stomach is talking to your mind, so everything should work out pretty well."

I like this theory and I agree that it is important for your brain to have ample time to react to what your mouth and stomach are up to, whether you're at home with a bowl of spaghetti or spending a long, enchanted evening in one of Keller's dining rooms.

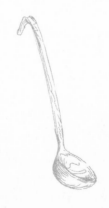

Thomas Keller's Yountville
Three Bean Salad

"Cooking is fairly simple when you think about it. Each technique is understandable and easily achievable if you really focus in on it," says Keller. "The difficulty, for me, comes when you are trying to do multiple techniques at once, and bring it all together into a dinner." So, while this recipe does have a lot of steps—Keller is nothing if not precise—none of them require special skill. And because it may be prepared a day ahead of serving, you can focus on following his meticulous instruction. To me, the most important is #21—taste and adjust seasoning and lemon juice. As with all of these chefs' recipes, make sure it pleases your own palate.

serves 4 to 6

FOR THE BEANS:

½ pound (1¼ cup) small red beans (such as Rancho Gordo's "sangre de toro"), rinsed

1 small carrot, peeled, stem removed

½ small red onion, peeled (reserve other half for the garnish)

1 large garlic clove, peeled, gently crushed

1 bouquet garni consisting of 1 fresh bay leaf, 6 parsley stems and 6 sprigs of thyme, tied together with kitchen twine

1 quart unsalted chicken stock (vegetable stock or water may be substituted)

2 teaspoons kosher salt

FOR THE GARNISH:

1 large yellow bell pepper

¼ red onion, sliced into ⅛-inch thick half moons
(about ½ cup)

3 red radishes about 1-inch diameter, stems removed, each cut into 8 wedges

1 large lemon, preferably a Meyer lemon

¼ pound yellow wax beans cut into 1½-inch pieces

¼ pound green beans cut into 1½-inch pieces

2-ounce piece ricotta salata cheese (Parmigiano Reg-
giano may be substituted but will have more fat)

FOR THE PARSLEY PESTO:

1 bunch flat-leaf parsley, large stems removed,
rinsed and drained well, coarsely chopped

1 small clove of garlic, peeled

¼ cup extra-virgin olive oil

¼ cup water

1 teaspoon salt

1. Preheat oven to 350°F.

2. Place beans, carrot, ½ red onion, garlic clove and bouquet garni in a small (2 qt) saucepan.

3. Add 1 quart of chicken stock, place over medium heat
and bring to a simmer.

4. Once simmering, skim off any impurities that rise to
the surface, cover with a tight-fitting lid and place in the
center of the oven.

5. Cook the beans in the oven for 2½ hours or until tender and creamy.

6. Once the beans are cooked, season with 2 teaspoons kosher salt and allow the beans to cool in the liquid. (Note: these beans may be cooked a day ahead of time.)

7. While the beans are cooking, place the yellow pepper on a small cookie sheet lined with aluminum foil and bake in the oven for about 30 minutes. Remove from oven and wrap the pepper loosely in a pouch of aluminum foil, seal and allow to steam for about 15 minutes or so.

8. While the pepper is steaming, combine the sliced red onions and radish wedges in a medium mixing bowl.

9. Finely grate the zest from the lemon (a microplane is perfect for this) and add to the bowl.

10. Squeeze the juice of the zested lemon through a strainer and combine in the bowl with a pinch of salt and allow to marinate.

11. Bring 2 quarts of water to a rapid boil in a saucepan and add 4 tablespoons of salt.

12. Fill a medium mixing bowl with about two parts cold water to one part ice.

13. Place the yellow wax beans and the green beans in the boiling salted water and cook for 2 minutes or until tender.

14. Once cooked, strain the green beans into a strainer and immediately plunge the beans in the ice water to stop the cooking process.

15. After the beans have been shocked, remove them from the ice water, drain well and add them to the marinating radishes and onions.

16. Remove the pepper from the foil pouch and carefully peel off the skin. Remove the stem and open the pepper up. Remove the seeds, rinsing if necessary.

17. Dice the roasted pepper into ½-inch pieces and combine with the marinating vegetables.

18. Combine the parsley, garlic clove, olive oil, water and 1 teaspoon of salt in a blender jar.

19. Blend until smooth and creamy.

20. Drain the cooled beans and combine with the marinating vegetables and the parsley pesto.

21. Adjust seasoning with salt and freshly cracked pepper. Acidity may be adjusted with more lemon juice if desired.

22. Transfer the bean salad to a serving bowl or platter.

23. Garnish the salad at the last minute with slivers of ricotta salata shaved on a mandoline or vegetable peeler.

24. Serve at room temperature.

Adapted from Thomas Keller.

Andrea Reusing's Warm Asparagus Salad with Soft-boiled Eggs

This is another of Reusing's wonderful salads that includes simple directions for homemade croutons. If you're really a carbophobe, I suppose you could omit them. But I think the better challenge is to make them without snacking on them before the salad gets to the table.

serves 4

4 large eggs, room temperature

Kosher salt

1 small clove of garlic

⅓ cup plus 2 teaspoons extra-virgin olive oil

Zest of 1 lemon

2 thick slices of country bread, crust removed, torn into rough 1-inch pieces

1½ pounds of asparagus, tough ends snapped off, cut into 2- to 2½-inch pieces

Small bunch fresh chives, cut into 2-inch lengths (½ cup)

½ cup flat-leaf parsley leaves

Freshly ground black pepper

1. Preheat the oven to 400°F. Fill a medium pot with water and bring it to a boil over high heat. Gently add the eggs with a spoon and simmer them over medium heat for 6 to 7 minutes—you want the yolks runny but without liquid whites. Transfer the eggs to an ice bath for 30 seconds; then remove.

2. Bring a fresh pot of generously salted water to a boil. Blanch the garlic clove for 30 seconds and remove with a slotted spoon. Reduce the heat to low until it is time to cook the asparagus.

3. Mince the garlic finely and transfer it to a small bowl. Stir in ⅓ cup of the olive oil and the lemon zest and set aside.

4. Toss the bread pieces with the remaining 2 teaspoons olive oil and a pinch of salt. Spread the bread out on a baking sheet and toast it for 5 minutes, until golden brown but still soft and chewy in the center. Peel the eggs and cut them crosswise into thick slices.

5. Bring the water back to a boil and blanch the asparagus for about 1 minute, until tender but still bright green. Drain the asparagus well, transfer it to a warm serving bowl and toss with 3 tablespoons of the garlic-lemon oil, the herbs, and salt and pepper to taste. Arrange the eggs and croutons on top. Drizzle with additional garlic-lemon oil and season it all, especially the eggs, with additional salt and pepper.

Adapted from Andrea Reusing.

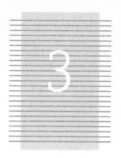

EAT THE WAY YOUR FAMILY DID

D URING OUR CONVERSATIONS, several chefs lovingly called out their parents who were not good cooks. To preserve the peace at his family's next holiday gathering, I won't name the chef who said of the woman who gave him life: "She can screw up cold cereal."

Another chef explained that both of his parents were world-renowned surgeons, so meals at home were handled mainly by babysitters who heated frozen dinners in the microwave for him and his siblings. On the rare night when his mom would cook, it was often a specialty they called "Desert Chicken." You'll never make it, but here's the recipe: "She would take chicken breasts, put them on a sheet pan with oil, put it in a cold oven, and turn it to three fifty. She would put rice in water, turn that on, put carrots in water, turn that on; then she would go upstairs and take a bath. Whenever she came down is when dinner was ready. By then, the chicken was screwed, the rice was a mess, and the carrots had turned to particles."

Future chefs who grow up like this start cooking out of self-preservation. But many more cited the way their parents or grandparents cooked and ate at home as the basis for their most healthful eating habits today. Here's what previous generations did right, and what inspires their chef progeny to eat well today.

Lesson 11: Smart chefs' parents cooked without processed convenience foods

"I was one of the lucky kids—I have a Greek and Sicilian mother," says Michael Symon. The owner of three metro Cleveland restaurants rarely ate out as a child. As a result, he benefited from a mostly Mediterranean diet at home: "A lot of greens, vegetables, meat, and fish. My father is Eastern European, which is another kind of food family—sausages, pierogies, stuffed cabbage."

As someone with forebears from Kiev myself, I have to say that those Eastern European delicacies are not exactly spa cuisine. But Symon points out that "everything was made from scratch, which I think is the biggest factor in staying fit. I'm a firm believer that all this packaged stuff Americans are buying up in gobs is making them fatter. When my grandfather wanted pie, he made a pie." His father's father, he adds, is ninety-four years old. "Healthy as a horse, lives on his own, golfs three days a week in the summer and bowls three days a week in the winter."

Today, Symon and his wife, Liz, cook at home often. Like the elder Symons, he reaches for real foods, not butter substitutes or any other supposedly healthful imitators (he shuns even turkey "bacon" as a processed impostor). Symon was particularly passionate and emphatic on this point, but many chefs felt the same: Eat real food. Food like previous generations ate—food made from ingredients that grow and eventually rot, not those that are manufactured and stick around unchanged through several presidential administrations even when exposed to the air.

The man with the pig tattoos still puts together the kind of balanced plates his mom did: "I love meat—it's my Midwestern upbringing," says Symon. "We do eat meat often, but we also eat a ton of vegetables and a lot of grains—quinoa and farro." Roasted beets are a frequent vegetable, and a favorite dinner, lifted from a houseguest's recipe, is chicken thighs with kale and potatoes, cooked in one pot. (The recipe follows.)

Lesson 12: They sought out great ingredients—and used them wisely

"My mother was very passionate about good food and good ingredients," says Alex Guarnaschelli. "I would joke that my mother would do the grocery shopping and *then* my parents would pay the rent."

I don't think anyone should endanger their mortgage for groceries, but her family had the right idea: Make wholesome food a priority. While wholesome and homemade doesn't necessarily mean fancy, buying more fresh, organic vegetables, fruits, fish, and meat may mean your grocery bill will go up. This is where it helps to borrow some restaurant chef behavior: Waste nothing. If you're going to invest more in quality ingredients, get as many meals as you can from them. (More on this in Chapter 6: Eat In Often.)

Even though preserving techniques like pickling, curing, and jarring feel old-fashioned today, Marcus Samuelsson argues that, "to truly be modern and contemporary, we have to know the past." As kids in Sweden, he and his two sisters would spend part of the autumn pickling vegetables and making jam with his grandmother and mom. "That wasn't work; that was fun; that was how we got together," he recalls. "Fall was plums and apples. Then mushrooms. I was having a good time, playing soccer with apples, throwing them at my sisters and cousins. Then cooking them with Grandmother. It sounds very old-school, but I grew up that way. Americans throw away one-third of our food today. That is not the way to move forward." I have to agree with him. While I'm not prepared to go full-on pioneer woman—freezing keeps food nicely too—I love the idea of a future where we all buy better-quality food, waste less of it, and are better fed and healthier for our efforts.

Lesson 13: They knew where their food came from

"My grandfather had an amazing green thumb," recalls Sueños chef-owner Sue Torres. "He took incredible pride in it. I mean, the grandkids could get away with a lot, but we didn't play ball around the garden, because that would be big trouble—you know, God forbid a ball should find its way into Grandpa's garden." This was her mother's side of the family, Italian and based in Bay Shore, Long Island. "The Italian side of my family was big into gardening, fishing, crabbing. We would bring a bridge table down to the marina with chairs and a deck of cards. The bait for the crab was chicken. My grandfather made his own crab nets, and we had a killie trap. Once we had some crabs, then we would go fishing—a big family affair in the summer."

A visit to Torres's other grandmother, who was Puerto Rican

and lived in Corona, Queens, sometimes meant a trip to the slaughterhouse. "My sister and I would call it 'the petting zoo,'" she says, laughing. "We would play with the little animals." While this struck me as surprising for a New York City borough in the 1970s, Torres points out that it wasn't at all odd in that community, with its many immigrants who had grown up in rural areas. Back on the farm in Puerto Rico, "She would go out, pick up a chicken, kill it, clean it, and start making dinner."

It is not as if Torres is catching her own crabs and slaughtering her own chickens. But the same attitude is easily adopted, without the hassle of a fishing voyage or trip to a slaughterhouse. (Note to Manhattanites: Would you even know where to find an abattoir, now that the meatpacking district is inhabited by fashion designers?) These days a big part of her job is working with purveyors to get the best ingredients. "That goes back to my Italian heritage—you have to have the best possible ingredients to make a great dish." It remains good advice: Buy the best you can. Look for local fish, meats, dairy, and eggs at your grocery and spend some time browsing the farmers' market.

But what came naturally to our grandparents can be both inspiring and daunting today. I would love to be the sort of cook who can prowl the market for what's freshest and looks most delicious, composing a meal in my head as I go. Ted Lee, despite being an expert recipe writer, is sympathetic. "My problem is I want everything, and I'll spend a hundred and twenty dollars and have nothing that goes together," he says. "I prefer a script." His coauthor and brother, Matt Lee, on the other hand, is one of those roamers who says, "The best-looking vegetable is the one I'll design a menu around. That's usually the way dinner begins." Try this, as he does, when you're not cooking for guests. "I prefer when the stakes are low," says Matt. "When it's just me and my wife, I swing for the bleachers a little bit. This is an opportunity to experiment."

It's understandable if none of this comes instinctually. Many of our parents were straight out of the canned-vegetable generation. The Lees had two parents who cooked; their father, they recall over our lunch together, was raised in a home with a big vegetable garden, and their grandmother and mother pickled. "But when we were growing up he made this chipped beef with artichoke hearts, remember?" says Ted.

"He used Buddig packaged deli beef that you shred," adds Matt.

"With canned artichoke hearts . . ."

"And the binder was cream of mushroom soup."

"Anyhow," says Ted, "it was delicious."

Lesson 14: They used meat sparingly, and kept portions modest

Wolfgang Puck's mother was a hotel kitchen chef in Austria, but at home "we ate very simple: noodles, salad, things from the garden," Puck remembers. "Very little meat, because it was expensive. Twice a month, maybe, we would have Wiener schnitzel." For the same reason, their portions were smaller than what most Americans today are used to. "When we cooked a chicken it was for six people." Not by coincidence, he says, "There were no big, fat people in the village where I grew up."

He can afford to eat whatever he likes now, but those early decisions made out of necessity inform how he eats to this day: He doesn't eat a lot of meat, preferring fish. When he does order a steak, he'll often split one eight-ounce portion with his wife. You don't need a lot of meat, he says, and, "You don't have to fill the plate."

I should add here that I don't believe having food be prohibitively expensive is a good way to cut down one's consumption. But meat in contemporary America has become perhaps too affordable, owing to shameful factory farming methods and animals confined to feedlots. It's worth it to pay extra for well-raised meat without added hormones and antibiotics, and if the upshot is that you're inclined to stretch it into a couple more meals by eating smaller portions, so much the better.

A little chicken story: After a disappointing corrupt-file experience at the computer fix-it shop, I was seeking solace and dinner makings in the nearby Chelsea market, with its Italian specialty grocer, excellent produce mart, and heritage-breeds butcher where the meats are laid out as if in a Tiffany jewel case. I asked for a small chicken, to roast for three people.

The man behind the counter—if his poultry was from old breeds, he was that new breed of tattooed hipster butcher—weighed it and told me the price. I flinched.

"Really?" I asked, and instantly felt a little shame at hearing my own accusatory tone. I wanted to add, "I'm not one of those people who expects to pay pennies a pound for factory-farmed chicken." But this was a very dear chicken.

He became gently defensive: "It's a red cockerel, very delicious. Very chickeny." I nodded and, somewhat shamed, paid for my little bird while listening to the internal monologue I'd inherited from my thrifty ancestors. *Very chickeny? So what should it taste like?* I later asked my mom what she was paying for well-raised chicken in Los Angeles. When I told her what I had paid, she said, reliably, "For that money it should have puckered up and kissed you."

You can bet that I treated that chicken with care. I massaged butter into its skin like a suntan lotion jockey at a posh hotel pool and roasted it with lemon and herbs in its cavity. I made stock from the neck and carcass, sliced white meat for sandwiches for my son and me, used the dark meat for tacos one night, and kept the rest in the refrigerator for a few days with my husband picking off a drumstick and wings.

You know what? When I stopped to consider what I've paid for a single-portion roast chicken dinner in a nice restaurant, I have to admit to you and to my tattooed butcher that this chicken was actually a good buy. And, yes, very chickeny.

Lesson 15: They didn't have dessert after every dinner

Although he was the youngest chef to earn the prestigious Meilleur Ouvrier de France certification in pastry, Jacques Torres did not grow up surrounded by desserts. As in many French families, postmeal sweets weren't a big part of typical dinners. "My mom would do dessert from time to time, but that was a special occasion," he recalls. More often dessert for Jacques and his brother was fresh fruit, abundant in the south of France, or a *petit suisse*, a fresh cheese with a similar consistency to yogurt, sold in individual containers. "She would put that on a plate with a little bit of sugar and a couple of strawberries mashed with a fork. That was a great dessert." Still is, if you can find it in your local store.

Michael Psilakis, raised by Greek parents in Long Island, New York, says, "We ate dinner together as a family for the first twenty years of my life, and dessert was a special thing. Mostly we had fruit after dinner; if we were watching TV, we would eat watermelon. My mother kept a bowl of fruit on the table. If you were walking by, looking for a snack, it was in front of you," he recalls. When he began losing weight, he remembered that. "It's a trick of suggestion, since whatever is in front of you is what you'll grab. If you have those grapes or berries or apples on the table that you pass constantly, you're sending a message to yourself: This is what you should be eating."

Another good trick from Sue Torres's family: The Sunday dinners she remembers were often a salad and pasta with meat—meatballs, sausage, braciola—and before dessert was served, fennel. "Grandma would bring out the fresh fennel with nuts and figs and say, 'It's good for your digestion.' Yeah, but with everything I just ate, is it really going to help?" She laughs. "But I love fennel."

I shared this idea with my son, who is often in a race to get to dessert. Telling him this was an Italian family tradition (my mother's father was half-Italian) made it appealingly exotic. So we tried it, and it helped that he liked the flavor. We don't serve a fennel course with the same regularity that Torres's family might have, but it is a nice pause before the end of a meal. I recommend it: Eat fennel. Okay, it doesn't have to be fennel, though many more people than Torres's grandma believe it is beneficial to digestion. If you don't like fennel, pause with a different vegetable. But choose a crisp, refreshing one that you can serve raw. Enjoy it, and the space it creates before dessert.

Lesson 16: They gave thought to the food they ate and served

"Our whole lives were centered around what we were going to eat next," says Portland chef Naomi Pomeroy of her bohemian upbringing in Corvallis, Oregon, in the 1970s. "My family was doing everything short of milling their own flour, almost. We didn't have a lot of money, but we had a garden and we ate out of it." Pomeroy's mother, who had been raised in a "boiled ham and iceberg lettuce" household, later lived in

France and taught herself to cook. As a result, the way of life she created for young Naomi "was focused around food. That was what we did for entertainment."

Living this way today takes time and effort. Is it possible to have a job and a family, and always be planning what you're going to eat? Probably not. But even a little planning helps: Buying apples that you intend to eat as a snack, and then actually remembering to put them in your bag when you leave for the day. Making enough extra dinner to have some lunch left over. Putting some forethought into cooking, rather than ordering takeout or heating up convenience foods, is simply better for one's diet.

"The more you cook at home, the more your lifestyle and health are going to tend to the good side," says Mark Bittman. His own mom "cooked mediocre housewife food of the fifties and sixties. But I started to cook when I was very, very young. So I started eating well young."

Note to myself: If a kid in 1950s Manhattan could pull a decent meal together, surely I can. I can't do it every day, but I can devote time on the weekend to shopping, cooking, and prepping a few things for the week ahead, including double portions of meals that will be lunch for me at work. If, like me, you are an obsessive reader and clipper of recipes that never get made, let us vow together that we will not fantasize about someday meals, but actually take those clippings to the store and plan to prepare and eat the food that inspires us.

Lesson 17: They didn't have hang-ups about carbs

As a boy, restaurateur Joe Bastianich ate most of his meals at Buonavia and Villa Secondo, the Queens restaurants that his mother, Lidia, and father, Felix, owned. (Lidia had worked in restaurants as a teenager, including a stint in a bakery run by the actor Christopher Walken's father. Knowing this may not improve how you eat, but it makes me happy to share it with you.) But there was always Sunday supper at home, with mom or grandmother behind the stove. Joe and his siblings, he says, "grew up in a house where the whole day was centered around what you're eating. We woke up at six a.m. to the smell of the first burning onions, because there was a fresh pot of consommé made. The amount of time spent talking about, and shopping for, and eating food was very different from what my friends experienced, which was maybe Hamburger Helper."

Instead, the Bastianich family was enjoying "roasted chicken and potatoes made in a cast-iron pan in the oven. Sauerkraut with pork and sausages, a typical dish from Trieste, Italy, where we're from. Or jota, a sauerkraut-and-kidney-bean soup. Seafood risotto. Tortellini *in brodo*. Always a lot of pasta." How did they manage it? For one, their portions were as traditional as their recipes: Italians don't consume pasta from a trough-size bowl the way some Americans do.

Some years later, in his thirties, Bastianich battled with his weight. When he remade himself as an athlete, the dishes from childhood became crucial building blocks of a healthy diet. He still eats pasta frequently, but now it fuels marathon or triathlon training sessions. Today, after a sixty-pound weight loss, he says, "My grandmother thinks I've lost too much weight. All she does is try to feed me."

Joe Bastianich's Spaghetti Pomodoro

This is a traditional sauce that is delicious straight up, or used as the base for Joe's scoglio, a shellfish pasta, which follows. Used alone, the pomodoro coats a pound of spaghetti very lightly. Double the recipe to have some extra, and then store ½-cup portions in freezer bags for convenience.

serves 6 as a pasta course or side dish

FOR THE SAUCE:

¼ cup olive oil

4 garlic cloves

28-ounce can whole Italian tomatoes

Salt and freshly ground pepper to taste

1. In a medium saucepan, warm the oil over medium heat. Crush the garlic cloves, remove the papery skin, add to the oil, and cook until fragrant and golden brown, about 1 to 2 minutes.

2. While the garlic cooks, pour the tomatoes into a bowl. Squeeze with your hands to break them up. Once the garlic is browned, add the tomatoes and any accumulated juices to the saucepan. Simmer over low heat for 45 minutes, adding water as needed to keep the sauce from becoming too thick. The sauce should be a rich red color. If it turns brick red, it's too thick. Season with salt and pepper to taste.

FOR THE PASTA:

3 tablespoons extra-virgin olive oil, plus more for serving

1 pound good-quality spaghetti, or spaghetti
chittara (chittara is long, square pasta; regular
spaghetti works just fine too)
Fresh basil leaves for serving
Grana Padano or other hard cheese (like Parmesan
or Romano), grated, for serving

1. Prepare pomodoro sauce.

2. While the sauce simmers, heat water for pasta. Add enough salt to make it as salty as seawater.

3. In a saucepan, heat up olive oil. Add pomodoro sauce (½ cup per serving) and simmer.

4. When the water comes to a full boil, add the pasta. Two minutes before the pasta is ready, remove the pasta from the water and add it to the pomodoro sauce. Cook the pasta in the sauce until tender, allowing it to absorb the flavor and color of the sauce. Add a little pasta water if needed to keep the sauce liquid. Serve with a drizzle of olive oil. Garnish with basil leaves and grated cheese.

NOTE: To turn pomodoro sauce into oreganata sauce, add 1 teaspoon dried oregano (preferably Sicilian) and several additional sprigs of fresh oregano to the pomodoro while it simmers. Remove sprigs before serving. To make arrabiata sauce, add hot pepper flakes to basic pomodoro sauce and simmer.

Adapted from Joe Bastianich.

Joe Bastianich's Scoglio

serves 4 as a main course

2 tablespoons olive oil, plus more as needed

8 medium-size scallops

8 medium head-on shrimp, peeled and deveined

2 fresh oregano sprigs

2 fresh thyme sprigs

Salt and freshly ground pepper to taste

8 mussels

8 clams

½ cup dry white wine

½ cup pomodoro sauce, as needed

1 pound spaghetti

1. In a large sauté pan, over medium-high heat, warm the olive oil. Cook scallops until golden brown on each side, about 1 to 2 minutes per side. Set aside. In the same pan, sauté shrimp just until they turn pink. Remove. Cut off the shrimp heads and add the heads back to the sauté pan along with 1 cup water, oregano, and thyme. Simmer for 10 minutes, scraping the bottom of the pan with a spatula to release any caramelized brown bits. Season the broth with salt and pepper to taste. Add mussels to the pan, along with a splash of olive oil, and cover with a lid. Remove mussels as soon as they open, about 2 to 3 minutes. Set aside. Repeat with the clams. Once the clams are open, about 10 minutes, remove and set aside. Remove the shrimp heads.

2. Cook pasta according to package instructions. While the pasta is cooking, strain the broth through a sieve set over a large bowl. Add the broth back to the pan, adding the white wine. Simmer over medium heat to cook off the wine. Add the scallops back to the pan, along with the pomodoro sauce. Add shrimp and a little more pomodoro sauce. Two minutes before the pasta is done, remove the pasta from boiling water and add to the sauté pan, stirring to coat with the sauce. Add more pomodoro sauce or pasta water as needed. Continue cooking the pasta in the sauté pan for another 2 minutes. Fold clams and mussels into the pasta. Serve immediately.

Adapted from Joe Bastianich.

Michael Symon's Chicken Thighs with Kale, Inspired by Lo

Symon nicked the idea for this recipe from pal Laurence Kretchmer, who is Bobby Flay's business partner. It has since become a favorite in my family too. Marcona almonds are milder and softer than typical almonds, which you may substitute.

serves 4

> 8 bone-in, skin-on chicken thighs, each about 5 to
>   6 ounces
> Salt and freshly ground pepper to taste
> 1 tablespoon olive oil
> 1 small red onion, thinly sliced
> 3 cloves garlic, thinly sliced
> 2 Fresno chilies, sliced in rings (substitute jalapeños
>   if you can't find Fresnos)

2 bunches of kale, roughly chopped
½ cup marcona almonds, roughly chopped
1 bay leaf
Zest and juice of 1 lemon
½ cup parsley leaves

1. Season thighs liberally on both sides with salt and pepper.

2. Warm the olive oil in a Dutch oven over medium heat, and brown thighs, skin side down, for 3 minutes per side. Place the chicken thighs on a plate.

3. Add onions, garlic, and chilies to the Dutch oven and sweat until translucent, about 4 minutes. Add kale, bay leaf, and 1 cup water. Salt liberally and bring to simmer. Place the chicken on top of the kale, skin side up, and place in 375° oven, uncovered, for 20 minutes, until chicken is cooked to internal temperature of 165°. Remove from oven and top with lemon zest and juice, almonds, and parsley.

Adapted from Michael Symon.

BEHIND THE LESSONS:

Sang Yoon's *Bubbe*

The birth of a restaurant is, in its own way, thrilling. Sang Yoon's Lukshon in Culver City, California, was not yet two weeks old when I ate there with friends, having earlier toured the place with its proud-papa chef-owner. On a February afternoon, Yoon showed me behind the scenes, where nothing was left to chance. He arranged for the water there to be filtered four different ways, depending on whether it is used to drink, wash dishes, become ice cubes, or rinse the stemware so as to not interfere with the taste of the cocktails. He revealed a remarkable system that he developed for serving wine on tap. Besides keeping air from touching the product until the minute it is drawn into a glass, his method is both less expensive and more ecologically sound than using bottles; I believe every restaurant should adopt it. He pointed out the sous vide machine, where beef for a spicy Malaysian curry rendang is cooked for forty-eight hours to render it "superdecadent, rich, and fatty. You'll try it tonight," he promises. I did; and it was.

Nothing was without a story. The menu is a showcase of modern takes on Southeast Asian cuisine, hitting many of the spots he traveled to with his father, a newspaper publisher. When I admired the cut-wood designs on the walls over the banquettes, he told me that they were laser-cut to precisely mimic swaths of vintage Chinoiserie wallpaper. Then there is the unlikely name. Lukshon means "noodle," which may not seem odd, as there are noodles on the menu—except that it means noodle in Yiddish. Sang is a lot of things—chef, athlete, entrepreneur, first-generation Korean-American—but Eastern European Jew isn't one of them.

"It's because of my *bubbe*," he says, using the Yiddish word for grandmother. He explains: "I had lost all my grandparents by age four. When I was in kindergarten my family met a woman who had grandkids in my class. She was a Jewish lady with flaming red hair and raspy voice who lived on Fairfax Avenue. When she found out I had no grandparents she instantly—no swearing-in ceremony—declared herself my grandmother. And it wasn't just lip service. She had twin granddaughters, and everything they did, I did. She made no distinction between those two girls and me. The name 'Lukshon' is an homage to that."

Besides being exceedingly generous to a boy who was a stranger, she was also, says Sang, an incredible cook. "Completely untrained, pure instinct. She was the first person to illustrate for me the difference between ordinary and Very Special. When she made chicken soup she would put in a beef rib bone to add more flavor, essentially cheating. Her neighbor would make us soup, and she'd say, 'Her soup, it tastes like the chicken sat next to the pot.' She was a massive influence on me. She taught me how to make gefilte fish from scratch. We made kreplach together. I'd say, 'Hey, these are like wontons!'

"What I found amazing is that Jewish and Korean cultures have so many parallels: the immigration, the work ethic, family values, emphasis on education and very similar pasts: The Jews worked together as families and opened small businesses. Fast-forward thirty years and it's all Korean store owners." Though he made his name in high-end burgers and beer at Father's Office, and built on it with Lukshon's luxe Southeast Asia cuisine, Yoon feels pride at the expansion and acceptance of Korean food in Los Angeles. "The food in K-town keeps getting better. It's interesting to see."

His *bubbe* died in 1999, but her influence is still evident. While it feels like this chef/scientist/inventor can do anything in his kitchen lab, when he wants a challah, he returns to his grandmother's old neighborhood. "I go to Beverlywood Bakery. That's the only good challah in town. I can't make that."

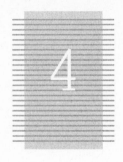

EAT BREAKFAST

MORNING PEOPLE ARE scarce in the restaurant world, and the question of breakfast seems to confound a lot of chefs. Should they eat it? Can they drink it? What happens if they ignore it altogether? And why is it (I've wondered this myself) that you most want a big breakfast the morning after eating a big dinner?

"Yes! What's that about?" asks Andrea Reusing, who has experienced the same weirdness. Knowing that you ate heavily the night before, should you give in to the unexplained desire for the full English breakfast, or put yourself on an austerity plan of green tea and grapefruit? Reusing is, like several of her colleagues, ambivalent about a morning meal. "I'm not a huge breakfast person, but I'll eat a bowl of cereal, or an egg, or fruit." Or just as easily, she says, "I can have a couple of cups of coffee and not need to eat until lunch." Nancy Silverton doesn't eat in the morning. Neither does Ted Lee, who says, "Everyone says you need breakfast for energy, but I've never experimented with that. I eat breakfast and I want to take a nap."

Melissa Perello is another breakfast skipper; she goes right to yoga or the green market or out to walk her dog, Dingo. All of those options sound reasonable to me, yet Perello expresses some doubts about whether they are the healthiest things she could be doing. Then she shrugs off her doubt. Perhaps she isn't starting every day with yogurt and wheat germ, but "I'm not eating Little Gem doughnuts." Hard to argue: Eating nothing until later must be better than starting the day with junk food. If you function well without a substantial morning meal, then eating one you don't want is just adding calories to your day.

Plenty of other chefs do eat breakfast, however, and many have habits worth adopting. Here are a few variations on their mornings.

Lesson 18: Smart chefs eat oatmeal

Unless they are on full carb lockdown, the most popular choice among chefs who eat breakfast is oatmeal. Nate Appleman became devoted to it as he dropped about a hundred pounds. It's useful to remember that oatmeal starts as a neutral base and you can either fancy it up with healthy accoutrements (fresh fruit, nuts) or you can use it as a sponge for brown sugar and render it as unhealthy as a box of rainbow-colored kiddie cereal. Resist that, and think like a chef: What else can I put on this canvas? Rick Moonen adds flax seeds, cinnamon, cayenne pepper, and just a drop of maple syrup. "Tastes like a Red Hot, and makes you feel really good," he says. "It gives me a little flush." Mark Bittman: "I like strong flavors: oatmeal with peanut butter or soy sauce. I'll have oatmeal with tapenade. Americans eat too much sweet stuff."

If you can remember to make the time (about thirty minutes), steel-cut oats are popular with chefs for a reason: They taste wonderful and have a more pleasing texture than rolled oats. But if you can't give it that kind of time, no matter. Sang Yoon contents himself with instant oatmeal at home too.

Lesson 19: They let breakfast shape the day to come

"Breakfast sets the tone for how I am going to eat for the rest of the day," says Sue Torres. She's lean and athletic and intense, and adamant about getting up and taking the time to eat something beneficial. "I feel like if I am just grabbing food on the go because I'm rushed, chances are it's going to be the same pace for lunch and for dinner. I stop and say, 'Okay, you have a busy day; you need to fuel up with the right stuff, the stuff that is going to carry you for three or four hours.'"

Torres always keeps Greek yogurt and fruit stocked, and sometimes blends them into a shake. Oatmeal or granola make regular appearances, and in summer she favors cottage cheese and cantaloupe—a combination that feels mildly retro to me, but that means it is probably due for a comeback. Usually, though, she goes heartier: eggs, bacon. "I've even had French fries, steak, and eggs for breakfast, because my Puerto Rican grandmother would make that every now and then for us. Oh, and plantains—just so much food it was ridiculous."

Susur Lee feels that a bowl of muesli is the best thing to both give energy and wake up the digestive system. "I eat this every morning," he tells me when we meet during one of his frequent visits to New York from Toronto. He wants to leave the breakfast table feeling satisfied, yet with an appetite for what will come during his workday. Since a lot of store-bought muesli is high in sugar, he makes his own, then has it ready to eat with yogurt and a drizzle of honey. His version, which contains nuts, oats, seeds, and two kinds of dried fruit, is a lot better-tasting than the boxed stuff. If you can find the ingredients in bulk, it's also cheaper. I made some and labeled the container "Mues-Lee." Feel free to copyright that, Susur.

Lesson 20: They find a breakfast that appeals, even when the idea of breakfast doesn't

"I never used to eat breakfast, but I've read how bad it is to skip it, because your metabolism never has a chance to get started," says Naomi Pomeroy. "So I started eating breakfast, a piece of wheat toast with my tea." Same deal across the country: Michelle Bernstein tells me, "In the last two years I've forced myself to become the kind of person who eats breakfast, since I started working out more." One of her preworkout breakfasts is a customized granola bar that she orders over the Internet. "You tell them online what ingredients you want in the bars and they make them for you. I have to have a say in everything I eat." Find them at Youbars.com.

When she isn't ordering from the iTunes of granola bars, she makes a fast protein-centered breakfast. "Something simple. I love peanut butter, so I try to get peanut butter in—I crave it when I wake up. Or I eat yogurt. Or a nice egg."

"A nice egg." That's precisely how she put it, adding that she doesn't eat bread in the morning. We should all face at least some days with "a nice egg." Get the best quality you can find, though those needn't come in brown shells or be tastefully speckled, like the ones Martha Stewart collects from the chickens in her yard. Go for those from free-roaming chickens, no antibiotics. However, no matter how nice the egg, it was a leap for me to follow Michelle's lead and omit the toast necessary to mop up the yolk. An egg by itself on a plate is a melancholy thing. It is the Morrissey of breakfasts.

Enter spinach. Inspired by chefs who eat vegetables in the morning (there are many), I discovered that sautéing a big bunch of fresh spinach—or, even better, mostly stemless baby spinach—can be done in the same pan in which you fry your egg. Canola spray, then spinach into the pan. After a quick stir to get all the leaves engaged in what's going on, crack an egg (or two) on top. Cover and cook over medium-low heat until the whites are opaque and the yolks still moving enough to become a sauce for the spinach when it all hits your plate. Pinch of flaky salt. That is a breakfast I could eat any day.

Lesson 21: They slow down and make breakfast a family meal

Because chefs are so often working during their children's dinner hour, breakfast is a way to sit down with the kids and bond over a meal, even if it is just a bowl of cereal and milk. Marc Murphy is happy to let his young son run breakfast each morning. Act one of his day often begins with his son pronouncing, "Daddy, let's go have breakfast!" How can you skip breakfast when you have that kind of invitation?

Breakfast with the family also motivates them to eat something at least as healthy as what they are feeding the kids. "I have breakfast with my daughter every day," says Alex Guarnaschelli. "It's an effort to encourage her to eat breakfast more than anything else. And because I think breakfast is important to get the metabolism going. We have fruit, oatmeal, yogurt with cereal—I'll sort of take my cue from what she'll have."

Wolfgang Puck will always sit down with his two young boys, even if he doesn't always share the same meal. "If they have oatmeal or cereal, I will," says Puck. "But I don't eat their pancakes or waffles."

On days off, Murphy does something more involved. "This weekend my daughter had a sleepover. I got up and made a broccoli-and-Parmesan frittata for them. They said, 'It's like pizza.' Kids love pesto, so I'll do green eggs. My daughter loves an English muffin with peanut butter. Good when you have a hangover, I find! Or we'll go to Chinatown; one of my favorite breakfasts is congee with dried scallops at Big Wong King, and steamed Chinese vegetables with oyster sauce."

I'm usually home at dinnertime, and can sit down with my son at that time. But breakfast with a kid in the house has made me think about eating better myself. It's hard to justify being both the parent who lectures on the importance of starting the day with a healthy meal—and also the harried woman racing to the first meeting of the day on nothing but a cup of coffee, who by eleven a.m. is falling face-first into a bagel.

Lesson 22: **They have a routine**

The morning, particularly when you're up early for exercise following a late night, is not the time to start pondering change.

Find what works and go with it. Thomas Keller alternates between a few standard breakfast choices. "Some days, two eggs, scrambled," he says. "Or a cereal with low-fat milk, usually Fiber One," to which he will add flax seeds and chia seeds (yes, the very same that make a Chia Pet grow; they have protein, healthy fats, and several minerals). "Once or twice a week, I'll do a protein shake with low-fat Greek yogurt and a banana," he says. "And every day for my beverage I'll do a probiotic, let me tell you the exact name of it—hold on…." He pads across the kitchen and comes back with the answer: Green Vibrance, which I later learn is a powdered blend of spirulina, seaweeds, edible grasses, vegetables, probiotic cultures and, well, some other stuff. (It's a long list.) "I'll have that with my vitamins, and then an espresso. That's mornings."

Ming Tsai also follows a routine, one that includes his own potent cocktail of healthy stuff. Into his blender goes a vanilla soy-based protein powder ("couple of tablespoons"), a banana, a tablespoon of green powder ("wheatgrass and all these good things for you"—it sounds similar to Keller's), a teaspoon of flax seeds, and some rice milk. The blended result is, he says, "a delicious, green *Star Wars*–looking shake."

The use of these pulverized nutritional powders strikes me as a bit of a departure from the whole-food/real-food philosophy to which most chefs subscribe. But there's an appealing hippie-science geek charm about blending bananas, flax, and so on that reminds me less of *Star Wars* and more of a scene from another film from the same year: Richard Dreyfuss mixing wheat germ, soya, and honey in *The Goodbye Girl*, while explaining to Marsha Mason, "My body is a temple . . . and I am worshiping it." Having a healthy, sippable, filling breakfast blend that you can toss together with one lobe of your brain still sleeping is a great idea. Ming has his alone, or accompanied by a piece of dense wheat-free, three-grain toast (Mestemacher is his brand of choice) with a slice of tomato and a few dots of olive oil.

When he began what became a 120-pound weight loss, Art Smith stuck with steel-cut oatmeal with berries and an egg-white omelet with vegetables. He named it the "Art Start," and put it on some of his restaurant menus. With his routine in place, he can now treat breakfast as a sort of reboot button, particularly if he goes off his usual diet on the previous day.

"Like last night, I had the most delicious Barack Obama burger at Spike's place," he tells me when we meet in Washington. (His friend Spike Mendelsohn's Good Stuff Eatery has a burger named for the president, topped with bacon, onion marmalade, Roquefort cheese, and horseradish mayonnaise.) "It was so delicious, with fries and a milk shake—I just had this food fiesta," says Smith, still delighting in this rare indulgence. "Then I got up this morning and started my journey back to wellness. You can still do these things, but you also have to keep going back to basic whole foods, to the miracles of oatmeal, the miracles of water."

Adding breakfast to a day that previously lacked it was a big part of both Nate Appleman's and Alex Stratta's routines and subsequent major weight losses. I've noticed that particularly among the guys who have dropped big numbers on the scale, having a regimen is everything. The same breakfast, the same lunch, a don't-miss workout appointment. It appears to be an antidote to the chaotic eating that once ruled their lives. Each wakes up to the whir of the blender. Stratta likes a mix of fresh berries, a banana, protein powder, soy milk, and coconut water. Appleman's recipe, which includes almond butter and honey, follows.

Lesson 23: Smart chefs don't let their coffee deliver loads of sugar or fat

Is it the hours they keep, or the easy access to the espresso machine? For whatever reason, chefs drink a lot of coffee. "My day always starts out with two cappuccinos, each with two shots of espresso. It's a ritual. It's part of waking up, like reading the paper," says Nancy Silverton. This is the big league. I myself idle way too high to take in that much caffeine, but Silverton tells me with a shot of pride, "I could drink an espresso falling asleep in bed."

Rick Moonen: three espressos. Naomi Pomeroy: an Americano. Colorado chef Lachlan Mackinnon-Patterson: cappuccino. Of the regular-coffee folk, Tom Colicchio sometimes drinks as many as four cups before he leaves the house. Donatella Arpaia admits to a time when she used to drink four to eight cups throughout a day.

The trouble with coffee isn't the coffee. It's what it can carry along with the coffee. Ted Lee and Matt Lee are both quite slim, but they noticed, says Ted, that "the main threat to our waistlines is the heavily sugared, half-and-halfed coffee we drink in the morning." Adds Matt, "I'm down to one cup. But I won't compromise on the sugar and the half-and-half." If you can't cut down on the number of cups, consider the formulation. Arpaia had a two-packets-of-sugar-per-cup habit. "With eight cups a day, that is a lot of sugar," she says. So she weaned herself off the stuff. "I went from two packets, to one packet, to half, to none. You train your palate that way." Colicchio too says he no longer automatically puts milk and sugar in his coffee.

I once believed that such a thing was impossible to do, until I observed that the way I was drinking coffee—with whole milk and sugar—tasted suspiciously like coffee ice cream in hot liquid form. I experimented with different roasts and beans until I found one I could love straight up. This was the most major step in retraining my palate to embrace tastes beyond sweet and salty—the two that my taste buds demand with the greatest frequency. There's so much more out there: bitter lettuces and twiggy Japanese green tea and tart plain yogurt (minus the jammy fruit on the bottom). Expanding the range of foods you can enjoy in their natural state is crucial to healthy eating. So while I'm up here on this particular horse, I'd like to add that I feel, as a new member of the black-coffee club, I've earned the right to issue a tiny manifesto: No flavored coffees; coffee *is* a flavor.

Lesson 24: They have creative coffee substitutes

One might imagine Joe Bastianich starts each day with the steaming screech of an espresso machine. But lately, he says, he's traded the caffeine in coffee for a piece (a small piece—not a bar) of dark chocolate. "It works," he confirms. "And it's more enjoyable."

I love this. Could I do it? I'm not sure. Hard to imagine sauntering into the conference room at work with a square of Scharffen Berger 82 percent while everyone else is nursing their coffee mugs. But I do love that Joe does this. After years of being overweight he is now insanely fit and can eat pretty much whatever he wants. If what he wants instead of coffee with sugar is a piece of chocolate, he has it and totally enjoys it. This is an important point that, I think, bears repeating when you get up and are too groggy to remember: Know what you *really* want to eat, and then enjoy it without guilt. Haven't we all, once in a while, eaten the breakfast we "should" eat and then, around about eleven a.m., sneaked in the treat that we were really craving?

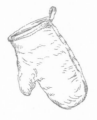

Nate Appleman's Breakfast Smoothie

The marathoning chef fuels up with this regularly. Tip: Peel and cut your bananas before freezing (store in plastic wrap). Yogurt without sugar is essential; the fruit and honey should provide enough sweetness.

serves 1 active person

COMBINE IN BLENDER:

- 1 frozen peeled banana, cut into 1-inch pieces
- ½ cup frozen peaches
- ¼ cup fresh blueberries
- ¼ cup plain yogurt
- 1 tablespoon almond butter
- 1 tablespoon honey
- 1 cup water
- Pinch of salt

Blend until smooth.

Adapted from Nate Appleman.

Susur Lee's Muesli

makes roughly 18 ¼-cup servings of muesli

- 1 cup raw oatmeal
- ½ cup raw almonds, chopped (or sliced)

½ cup raw walnut halves or pieces

½ cup raw hazelnuts

½ cup sunflower seeds

½ cup pumpkin seeds

½ cup dried cherries

½ cup raisins

Mix ingredients together and store in airtight container.

FOR SERVING:

1 tablespoon Greek yogurt

Milk or soy milk

Honey

Serve a portion (¼ to ½ cup) in bowl with Greek yogurt, a splash of milk, and a small trickle of honey.

Adapted from Susur Lee.

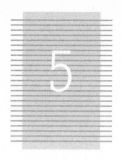

EAT BIG FLAVORS

"I'LL OVEREAT WHEN I don't feel satisfied—when I can't get those flavors I'm looking for," says Nancy Silverton. Her insight stands some conventional wisdom on its head: Many people think that, faced with something incredibly delicious, they won't be able to stop. But Silverton observes in herself a tendency to keep picking away at different things until her palate is happy. Might as well identify what that is and have it up front. For her, sometimes it's just a spoonful of caramelized onions or of small croutons freshly tossed with olive oil and salt, both of which she has handy when she's working behind the mozzarella bar at Osteria Mozza. "I love the crunchiness, the oiliness, the saltiness. It takes care of those cravings so I don't overeat."

The importance of eating food that delights your mouth shouldn't be understated. This is why you talk to chefs about eating lightly: They do not compromise flavor when they cut calories. A survey turns up a useful list of items—mostly kitchen staples, and a few ringers worth investigating—that crank up the flavor of a dish without adding much in the way of calories or excess fat. There are many more than what are listed here, but these items and techniques were the most frequently and enthusiastically mentioned.

Lesson 25: Smart chefs start with the best ingredients available to them

Thomas Keller is breaking it down for me. "Cooking is an equation: Execution + Ingredients," he says. "The best ingredients you can get will result in the best food you can cook—as long as you don't screw them up." He allows that there are other factors: individual skills, environment, equipment. But great ingredients, he feels, are paramount. He offers a good example of a dish that relies entirely on the strength of its ingredients, no technique: A tomato salad from very fresh, ripe tomatoes. "You've done that, right? Sat down to a meal like that? It's a really simple thing, and you go, 'My god, that's just incredible!' The tomatoes speak for themselves, you just cut them, put some great salt on them and some olive oil and vinegar and it's like, wow! There are four components there—tomatoes, salt, oil, vinegar—but, done right, when the tomatoes are amazing, it's compelling and impressive."

With truly wonderful ingredients you can, even lacking Keller's training, make something amazing. Buying the best you can has another benefit: It sustains the small farmers and other purveyors from which some of the finest products come, and puts corporate producers on notice that we won't accept tomatoes that more closely resemble High-Bounce Pinky balls. "That we have to do as a society anyway," says Keller, "support our farmers, our foragers, our fisherman, our gardeners."

Lesson 26: **They salt their food**

With your ingredients gathered, it's now time for technique. Here's an easy one: Put some salt on the food you are cooking. There are people who, on their doctors' recommendation, should avoid eating too much sodium. If this is you, take this section with a grain of . . . you know. But if you don't have a health reason to be concerned about salt, well, why are you being so stingy with it? "If you're eating Cheez Doodles and ramen cups you probably shouldn't be having salt any other time of the day," says Marc Murphy. "But if you're eating food that you've made yourself, don't be scared of the salt." Skip the sodium-enhanced processed stuff, and instead cook real food, seasoning it right.

Murphy is not alone in this philosophy. For flavor, salt is a miracle drug, according to *every single chef* with whom I spoke. "Bland food doesn't have to do with the quality of the ingredient, it has to do with seasoning it correctly," notes Keller. "If you take a scallop and don't season it at all, it tastes bland. You add a little bit of salt to it, and you go, 'This is an amazing scallop!'" Salt: It makes vegetables more vibrant; it makes chocolate less cloying . . . it puts the ape in apricot. Yet many pros feel that home cooks are woefully underseasoning their food.

"If you don't salt your pasta water before you cook it, the pasta's not going to taste good," says Murphy. "If you don't have it over the whole piece of protein before you sear it, [it's] not going to form a crust." Then he offers this challenge: Take a steak, cut it in half, season one side the way you normally do, and on the other side go crazy—put what you think is too much. "The second one, the one that you've seasoned properly—what I call 'seasoned with authority'—will taste better. Yet people are scared of seasoning. They say, 'Well, I have salt and pepper on the table if people want more.' It's too late—you cannot add salt to those cooked carrots and make them taste as good. It's got to be in the cooking. It brings the flavor out." By now he's a bit riled as he adds dramatically, "Don't. Be. Afraid."

Kosher salt is good for many tasks, from brining meats to seasoning vegetables. (For baking, use fine-grained salt.) If you want to get more involved than that, there are many others: red or black Hawaiian salts that may contain coral or lava, smoked salts, flavored salts (truffle—a Naomi Pomeroy favorite—or celery, vanilla, garlic, etc.), and salt blends, like Japanese salt with bits of seaweed. Few people rave about ordinary table salt, though it is the only one that is reliably a source of iodine, which your thyroid gland needs. The Lee brothers and many more cooks swear by flaky Maldon salt from the south coast of England, and I've since invested in a box. Save these pricier, toothier salts—French *fleur de sel* is another—for finishing a dish; don't dump them in your pasta water. Instead, make toast, melt some dark chocolate on it, and sprinkle a few flakes of Maldon over it. Not doing bread and chocolate today? Put a pinch on a slice of watermelon—if you take no other advice, try this. It will make you leap with joy.

One more thing: Keeping some salt handy in a little bowl or box to take pinches from will make you feel more like a chef. If you have ever struggled to measure a "pinch of salt" from your saltshaker, you'll fast understand why chefs don't use them.

When remembering the salt in savory dishes, don't overlook

its natural counterpart, black pepper, which has lost shelf space to all sorts of fancier cousins. Once a week Murphy mills some peppercorns in a coffee grinder and makes a 25-percent-pepper/75-percent-salt blend, which he keeps on hand for seasoning. "Get to be in love with black pepper again," advises Andrea Reusing.

Lesson 27: **They don't drop the acid**

Second only to salt, acid is a key component of what chefs know makes a dish pleasurable. Whether from vinegar, citrus juice, or verjuice (the juice of unripened grapes or other fruits), they rave about the brightness that acid gives a dish, especially as a foil for fatty foods. "Vinegar does the same thing as salt, which is it heightens flavor," explains Thomas Keller. "You don't want to taste either one—unless that's your goal, as in a scallop *au vinaigre*. When we make a sauce, we're using both salt and vinegar. Neither one do you taste, but the flavor of the sauce is heightened."

And yet for some reason home cooks—and cookbooks aimed at us—are less apt to consider acid as a way to improve flavor. "If you've followed a recipe and it didn't turn out quite so good, it probably needs salt and acidity," says Rick Moonen. Moonen loves lemon—the juice and the zest—to improve a dish. "If you want to brighten something up, try taking the zest off any citrus that catches your eye: lemon, lime, grapefruit, tangerine—all good. Those oils are amazing." He recommends a microplane, an über-sharp grater that I long resisted buying, until I caved and wondered what I had been waiting for. Get one; it will change your life.

Michael Psilakis, who uses an olive oil–lemon-salt-pepper

blend frequently, explains why acid is essential. "Acid helps us experience food on a palate at different times, so you have an evolution as opposed to a uniform flavor profile throughout the process of chewing. When you add acidity you experience the food as a sort of roller coaster, with peaks and valleys, which is a lot more fun than driving on a flat plane."

That lemon-oil blend added to a piece of grilled chicken or fish "will combine with the natural juices, and create a beautiful warm vinaigrette on the plate," says Psilakis. "The salad greens will soak up the juice, and you get to have the bitterness of the greens combine with the sweetness of the caramelization coming off the grill." Many more chefs extolled the combination of olive oil, lemon, and salt (with or without pepper). You don't really even need to be cooking to benefit from the combination. When he wants a fast lunch, Ted Lee will open a small can of tuna, liven it up with some good olive oil, vinegar or citrus juice, Maldon salt, and pepper, with pickles (another great use of vinegar) on the side. "We always have a lot of quick pickles on hand," says Ted. "Pickles dress up anything."

I adore pickles, from kosher sour dills to hot and garlicky kimchi to neon-colored Japanese oshinko. Guided by recipes from the Lees, Michael Symon, and Andrea Reusing, I've started making batches of "quick" pickles, those that are brined gently in the refrigerator and can be served within a few hours. I've done white radishes and red onions and even grapes in a rose-mary-infused brine (hat tip to the Lees on that). Where I get a bit nervous is with the fermented variety, for which you need to trust the brine to develop in a cool corner of a room over several days, a sort of controlled rot that unnerves control freaks like myself. (In quick pickling, the acid in vinegar does the work that the microbes formed during fermentation handle.)

"You have a fermentation fear. That's normal," Reusing tells me over lunch one day. Then she sets out to cure it. "What temperature is your apartment? Temperature is the critical thing: Keep it between sixty-eight and seventy-two degrees. It will bubble a little. You have to be willing to throw some stuff away until you get it right."

"How will I know if I should throw it out?"

"You'll know it's bad. It's going to be funky, and not in the good, Korean deli sense. You shouldn't be afraid. Do it! Do a white kimchee with baby turnips and green chilies and ginger. Really easy. Your kid will love it." Yes, my son loved the turnips. But unlike me, he didn't have the worry that I might have been growing something closer to penicillin than to a condiment. I'm not sure this will enter my weekly rotation of standards, but it's good to conquer a fear and have another trick in the arsenal.

As for which vinegars to stock, many quick pickle recipes call for white vinegar, but you wouldn't want to use that for most cooking. Lachlan Mackinnon-Patterson, chef-owner of Boulder's Frasca Food and Wine, believes a basic wardrobe should include, at minimum, a good red wine vinegar and a real balsamic.

Naomi Pomeroy is a fan of aged balsamic vinegar, a mellower acid, to add complexity to a dish. "A really good, thirty-year-aged, true balsamic," she explains. "Not some weird reduction of regular balsamic with caramel color." The real deal "is amazing. It adds acid, but sweetness, and a little of the umami flavor," she says, referring to the savory fifth taste. "Those are the things that are going to give you the most power." A thirty-year balsamic doesn't come cheaply, but consider investing: The concentrated flavor delivers a lot of zip with just a few drops. A cooking note: Acids can turn green vegetables brown; don't squeeze lemon on your spinach until you're ready to eat.

Lesson 28: **They employ oil strategically**

When considering acid's most frequent partner, olive oil, one should remember that oil of any kind has a lot of calories, all from fat. Everyone uses it, including people like Alex Stratta, who has pushed most other fats off the table to maintain his hundred-pound weight loss. "I refuse to cheat on olive oil," he says. "I won't give that up. I have to have some texture." But for some in serious shedding mode, olive oil may have to come under scrutiny. "People say, 'Oh, I'm just having salad,' and then they dump three hundred and sixty calories, a.k.a. three table-spoons of olive oil, on their plate," notes Alex Guarnaschelli. "By my calculations, that's one and a quarter Snickers bars. If I'm going to be on a diet and have that Snickers bar moment—where I have to have a Snickers bar—I don't want to have al-ready spent three hundred and sixty calories on olive oil. And I love olive oil."

While the oil-and-vinegar equation is common on salads, a great vinaigrette is a clever replacement for sauces on meats. "Typically, saucing involves items that are fattening," notes To-ronto chef Mark McEwan. "People use jarred barbecue sauces without realizing what's in there—they are laden with calories. Instead, do a horseradish vinaigrette, which you can put on fish, chicken, beef. It's a universal condiment. I think it's the new ketchup." (His recipe appears on page 184.)

Another reminder: Don't fry with extra-virgin olive oil, be-cause it can't take high heat without smoking and turning bit-ter. Use a neutral oil like canola to sauté food; then finish a dish with just a drizzle of extra-virgin olive oil or another flavorful, rich oil like walnut; you need only a little to get the taste. Bet-ter yet, cook with steam, then finish with oil. "When I cook vegetables—carrots, string beans, asparagus, corn, whatever—I always steam them," says Wolfgang Puck. "Then sprinkle some good olive oil on top with a little sea salt."

Lesson 29: They harness the heat of chilies

"Chilies help you feel more satisfied," offers Rick Bayless. "They fire your mouth on all cylinders." He also points to studies suggesting they can speed up your metabolism. "Chilies can be your friend if you're trying to lose weight." One of the easiest ways to get chilies into your life is with a can of chipotles in adobo, which are smoked, dried jalapeños in a vinegar-and-tomato broth. Bayless advises dumping the contents of an entire can in a blender, whirring, and using the resulting puree on "practically anything: soup, beans, or as a marinade for fish or chicken. Superdelicious." Another way: chop tomato, cilantro, green chili, onion, and garlic into a fresh salsa. "If there isn't some chili in a menu, you're leaving out a flavor and there's a hole." Andrea Reusing blends chili, garlic, and shallots into oil for a fast condiment.

Not just Mexican cuisine, of course, but also those of South America, Southeast Asia, India, North Africa, and China rely on the punch of chilies. During my brief swing through China in 2011, I became besotted with the bright red chilies used in Chengdu—some with great names like "facing heaven." There's a spice native to the region called a flower pepper (not a pepper at all, really, though it is sold in the States as "Sichuan peppercorns") that numbs your tongue a bit in a way that is at first unnerving, and then delightful.

Interestingly, when I ask Susur Lee (who hails from Hong Kong) about his favorite peppers, he reveals that even in some

Chinese dishes he reaches for the very hot (and Western-culti-vated) Scotch bonnets and habañeros. I find this sort of cross-cultural fusion not only freeing, but essential as a home cook who doesn't want to have to buy one-use-only ingredients to make a dish. There's no reason to hunt high and low for a spe-cific chili for your ma-po tofu, unless you find the search to be part of the fun.

Not surprisingly, Sue Torres of New York's Sueños is another chili proponent, who wants to win over those who fear them. "People say, 'Oh, I don't like spicy.' But not all chilies are spicy. A lot of them have fruity flavors, like raisin, cherry, or prune."

After our interview Torres asks whether I'd like anything to eat—her staff is starting to put out a family meal of chicken and rice. Earlier in the day I had met with Eric Ripert, and his no-eating-between-meals edict is still ringing in my ears. No, thanks, I say; I'm on my way home to make dinner. "Would you like some chilies?" she asks.

I take home a brown-paper-wrapped package of anchos (mild dried poblanos) and her directions for this easy sauce: Roast tomatoes, onions, and garlic and whirl in a blender with some toasted, soaked anchos and a little salt. Or, if you don't have the time or inclination to roast, try fresh tomatoes, onions, and cilantro.

Per her instruction, I toast the anchos in the oven. After about ten minutes I swing the door open to check on them, and am hit by a scent that is woody and chocolatey. They are done, so I drop them into a bowl with hot water to soften, then start searching for tomatoes and onions and cilantro. No, no, and no. I do have a can of peeled tomatoes, and some garlic. (Not the same thing, I know.) Since I'm going off the rails with this, I throw in some tangerine, raisins, cinnamon, salt, and pep-per. I spin it through the blender, warm the sauce, and serve it alongside poached cod and roasted sweet potatoes. (A sauce that strange you don't serve on top of the entrée.) But it's a total hit with both the kid and the husband. We dub it Found Items Mole, and it proves highly flexible, adding warmth and spice to several dishes throughout the week.

Lesson 30: They use fresh herbs

Dried herbs are undeniably handy, and you certainly shouldn't toss the collection you've probably amassed. (Though weeding them out every year or so isn't a bad idea.) But if you haven't bought fresh in a while, do. For encouragement, here's a mini-tutorial on herbs from Michael Psilakis:

"Herbs can be grouped in a very simple way, either savory or sweet. Savory (like rosemary, thyme, or sage) we want to cook with, and sweet (mint, basil, cilantro, dill) we want to add at the end. Savories will influence the flavors of the sauces or the marinades or the meats as we're cooking them, but you don't necessarily know they are in there. To braise lamb shanks we use rosemary, but there's also carrots, celery, onions, garlic, and cumin. So rosemary is in there, but it's just part of the depth of flavor.

"Sweet herbs are those that we're going to use in their natural raw state to brighten food up and get that herbaceousness. Sweet herbs create specific flavors that you're going to experience individually, which is very different. So if you're chewing something and then you hit a piece of mint you get that mint. Or that cilantro. That's the beauty of Mexican food or Asian food—all these spices and herbs right out there." A great example is a bowl of Vietnamese pho—noodles in broth with a little meat, topped with fresh, uncooked herbs like coriander,

Thai basil, and purple shiso. "I eat that a lot," says Susur Lee. "Having the herbs on top gives a great flavor."

Lesson 31: **They always have garlic handy**

"Garlic is the most magical ingredient to make something sexy," says Eric Ripert. I have to agree that it is sort of magical how it partners with olive oil one night and then with fresh ginger and soy sauce the next. Adds Alex Stratta: "I love garlic. Smothering something with roasted garlic gives a lot of bang for the buck." Rick Moonen seconds that, saying, "You can never have enough garlic." At home, Ming Tsai likes the shortcut of a prepared garlic oil that he uses to sauté spinach, broccoli, cauliflower, or Brussels sprouts. "My kids eat Brussels sprouts because of this flavor," he raves.

Fresh garlic is easy to keep on hand. But don't be a snob about the dehydrated stuff in the spice rack—employed creatively it can also elevate a dish. "I use garlic flakes and onion flakes to make 'everything-crusted' fish—you know, like an everything bagel?" says Moonen. "Sesame seeds, poppy seeds, onion, garlic, and salt. Put that on a piece of tuna and sear that. People love it. Serve with a red-pepper coulis—burn up a red pepper and puree it with some vinegar, salt, pepper. That's all you need. It's good."

Lesson 32: **They have favorite flavor tricks**

By nature, chefs are experimenters. They enjoy playing with flavor profiles different from the ones they work with all day in their restaurants. "I did a pork vindaloo the other day," says

Moonen, describing a venture into Indian flavors that are far from the clean seafood dishes for which he's known. "I boned out a pork shoulder and marinated it in my own tamarind paste with cinnamon and cardamom and cloves—so deep, so rich, so wonderful." But chefs also all have reliable flavors that they return to again and again. Here, a roundup:

- Coriander seeds, says Sue Torres. "Take a chicken breast, salt, and pepper; crush coriander seeds and crust the chicken in them. Pan-sear, slice it up, and serve on salad." It's just one step more than simply seasoning with salt and pepper, and the lemony fragrance of coriander seeds can refresh a familiar dish. (Coriander seed is not the same as fresh coriander, also known as cilantro.)
- "A bundle of thyme, marjoram, rosemary, or bay in a little sachet tossed into soups or stocks," says Melissa Perello. That will round out the flavor, adding notes that a single herb alone can't do.
- Herbes de Provence blended on fish, chicken, beef, roasted vegetables—almost anything, according to Eric Ripert. Using this classic French mix, which usually contains dried fennel, basil, thyme, savory, and lavender, "You can have food that is light, and has a lot of flavor," says Ripert, who, as a boy, used to harvest the herbs with his grandmother to dry and mix their own.
- Curry blends, according to Sang Yoon. Contrary to popular misconception created by jars of generic "curry powder," curry isn't a single spice, but a mix of several. There are countless variations, ranging from sweet to sour to hot. "Curry is so flexible; use

it on fish, shrimp, beef, chicken, vegetables. Make
a pot of rice, a curry dish, a salad—*boom*, done."

■ Fish sauce, per Naomi Pomeroy. "If you're not al-
lergic to fish, I swear you should be pouring that
all over everything. A couple of dashes in any soup,
instead of salt."

Her advice was a revelation to me. There is usually a bottle
of nam pla in my fridge, and it is usually seven-eighths full,
because I'll buy it once a year when I feel like making pad thai.
Pomeroy suggested that I could use it in recipes that are not
traditionally Asian to add depth of flavor, just as you might use
Worcestershire sauce. "It's a cleaner alternative. Just a dash—it's
amazing. Next time you make tomato soup throw it in there."
(Her recipe for tomato soup with fish sauce follows.)

A final thought about expanding your spice and condiment
library: You can happily get by with nothing but salt, lemon,
and olive oil to dress up a huge array of dishes. When you're
cooking from recipes, however, you're bound to be asked to use
some sauce or herb or spice that you've never owned, and for
that reason you may be inclined to skip making the recipe altogether. I know I've passed over recipes that called for too
many ingredients with an asterisk that took me down to the
bottom of the page for detailed purchasing instructions.

Case in point: Michelle Bernstein's recipe for tomato-water-
melon-feta salad, below, suggests a dried herb called za'atar in
the dressing. There are countless twists on watermelon salads,
and I felt it was important to try hers exactly as written. So off
I went to get za'atar. I live near three excellent grocers, but none
carried it. I had to go to a spice store twenty-four blocks away,
which might not sound like a lot if you live in one of those
cities where you can have a car, but was a major event on a

Sunday afternoon for me. Once I was there, however, za'atar was no longer exotic. It was on the shelf, plain as day: za'atar from Israel, from Jordan, from Lebanon. There was another with no country of origin on the label, so I bought that one, not wanting to play favorites. I was able to taste the recipe as Bernstein had intended it (it's subtle and refreshing, and my son drank the juice left in the bottom of his bowl), and, as a bonus, I now had a new toy in the box with which to experiment. So far, I've found it's good sprinkled on pizzas and in eggs.

As you accumulate new ingredients, try not to let the ones you like languish until the next time you make the exact recipes that demanded them in the first place. Think like a chef, and just mess around in the kitchen with that random spice, adding it to, say, sauces, pastas, eggs, chicken. When chefs talk about "ingredient-driven cooking," this is sort of what they mean: They don't use recipes, but let what's fresh, what's in season, and what's on-hand determine what is going on the plate. So you've got some chicken, and peas and zucchini are happening at the market, and look, there's your new jar of za'atar . . . go. The opposite is recipe-driven cooking, and if that's what you're more comfortable with, be grateful we live in the age of the search engine: Throwing "za'atar" into the database of a cooking Web site has given me ideas from za'atar aioli to spiced eggplant fries.

Lesson 33: They are not immune to the smoky charms of bacon

This is not the low-fat section any longer. But if we are to acknowledge that we are living in bacon-wrapped times, we should talk about the best way to use it, which is to say sparingly. Andrea Reusing is fond of the Southern tradition of flavoring turnip greens or collards with a knob of bacon or a smoked turkey wing. This is meat as a cooking tool, not as the main event, and you don't need a lot. Get the kind that is raised well and not full of so many nitrates that it glows in the dark. Reusing likes Benton's bacon, made in Tennessee and popularized in New York by Momofuku chef David Chang. "It's like a walk through the smokehouse."

Rick Moonen relies on it to perk up lentils. "Render out the bacon, get the fat going, put some onions in there, a pinch of ras al hanout [a Moroccan spice blend], put your lentils in there, water, simmer it—yee-haw!"

Melissa Perello will use the rinds from prosciutto, which have less fat than the flesh, in stocks or sauces, or in a braise. "We do use a lot of bacon at the restaurant and a lot of it gets recycled," says Perello. "We'll throw a big piece of raw bacon in with the beans. When the beans are cooked you end up with this beautiful knob of braised bacon, so sometimes a chunk of that gets used to flavor another dish. You're not getting the bacon, just this nice smokiness."

Vegetarian? Going low-fat? There are other ways to get a comparable flavor. "Smoked paprika," notes Matt Lee, "gives you that smoky profile in a way that doesn't add animal fat."

Lesson 34: They use water as a medium for flavor

"I love flavorful broths," says Alex Stratta. "Tamarind, lemongrass, lots of ginger, and garlic." Beginning with a base of water and aromatics, chefs create dishes with minimal fat, maximum taste. Perello suggests tossing the rind end of a Parmesan cheese into a vegetable broth. "Even though it's a cheese, you're not imparting a lot of fat, but you do get a lot of flavor."

"I use a lot of dashi," says Michelle Bernstein. Dashi is a Japanese stock of kombu seaweed and bonito flakes (dried, fermented, smoked tuna shavings—which, wow, doesn't sound so great as I write it but is—trust me—delicious in stock or on top of tofu and rice). As with fish sauce, I tended to relegate dashi to Asian dishes. But Michelle sees no reason not to cross boundaries, and treats it as a base for fennel, peppercorns, dill, and lemon zest, and then, adding olive oil, uses it to poach fish. "Then I reduce the broth and add vegetables and let the broth dry up so it gets really glaze-y. I put the vegetables on top of the fish—delicious."

What's interesting is how her restaurant cooking has lightened since she is herself eating lighter, broth-based meals. "I think there are only three or four dishes on my whole menu of twenty-five items that have butter on them now. I don't use heavy cream on but one dish. I used to think those things made food delicious—and they do! But they are not the only things."

Sue Torres will poach fish in water and white wine, using up scraps of onions, carrots, celery, garlic—"whatever you've got." Or leave out the wine and substitute coconut milk, adding a whole habañero chili for heat (don't accidentally serve the pepper). "Bring that stuff to a boil, reduce it down, then poach fish in that."

While many Americans are comfortable with that method for fish, Torres points out that in Mexico, it is just as common for beef or pork, which takes a lot of fat out and floats it away. "Cook the meat with some water, garlic, carrots, chayote [a summer squash], bay leaf, peppercorn, and a little epazote [a Mexican herb]. You skim the fat from the top, and shred the meat," she says. "Now you can take that roasted tomatoes, onions, and garlic and chipotle or ancho chili and mix it in with your beef, or pork, and you have a pretty healthy dish." A note on poaching and simmering: They are not the same as boiling. For these, keep the water between 130° and 185°F to cook food slowly and gently. Poaching liquid shouldn't roil at all, and simmering should have only an occasional bubble. Odd as it may seem, even sitting in water, food can dry out when boiled.

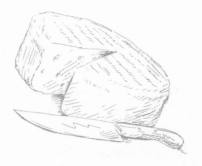

Sue Torres's Shredded Beef

This is easy and great for tacos, over rice, or cooled to room temperature and served on salad. Sue's ranchera is a perfect accompaniment—you will stop buying jarred salsas!

serves 10 to 12

> 5 pounds beef chuck roll (stew meat), cut into
>   2-inch–3-inch cubes
> ½ medium white onion, roughly chopped
> 1 carrot, peeled and roughly chopped
> 3 garlic cloves, peeled
> 1 bay leaf
> 1 ear of corn, roughly chopped
> 1 chayote or zucchini, roughly chopped

1. Place all of the ingredients in a large, heavy pot with enough water to cover. Bring to boil over high heat. Reduce the heat to medium. Cook until the meat is tender, about two hours.

2. Remove from the heat and carefully strain through a colander set over a large bowl. Reserve liquid if you desire for another use, skimming the fat before use. (Broth is great for soups or stews.)

3. While the beef is still warm, shred with fork. Serve with salsa ranchera (recipe below).

This can keep in the refrigerator for 4 to 5 days.

Adapted from Sue Torres.

Salsa Ranchera

makes 1 quart

6 (about 3 pounds) beefsteak tomatoes
½ small white onion, skin removed, cut into quarters (no more than 3 ounces in weight)
2 garlic cloves
2 jalapeños

1. Heat a griddle or comal (400°F) over high heat. Place the tomatoes, onion, garlic, and jalapeño on the hot griddle and cook until blackened. Turn the vegetables on the griddle every couple of minutes for even cooking. The garlic and jalapeño will be ready before the tomato and onion. Depending on the size of your griddle, you may need to do this in batches. Once each vegetable has a nice blackened char on all sides, remove from the heat.

2. Let cool to room temperature before pulsing in food processor for a couple of seconds, to a chunky consistency. Do not overprocess the salsa; it should be coarse, not smooth. Season with salt to taste.

This can keep in the refrigerator for 3 to 4 days.

Adapted from Sue Torres.

Sue Torres's Grilled Vegetable Tacos with Cilantro Pesto

Serranos, called for here, have a fair amount of heat. Jalapeños are a milder substitute. Torres layers the flavors: During the grilling, then with the cilantro "pesto" and finally the pico de gallo.

serves 6

FOR THE PESTO:

- 1 cup packed fresh chopped cilantro leaves and stems
- 1 garlic clove, thinly sliced
- ½ cup oil (Sue likes a blend that is about 25 percent olive, 75 percent corn—you can eyeball this)
- ⅛ cup toasted pine nuts
- salt

1. In a blender, combine the cilantro, garlic, and half the oil. Pulse several times until it starts to purée. Add the pine nuts, and pour the remaining oil in slowly, pulsing until it is just blended, not liquefied. Season with salt to taste

2. Set aside for immediate use with the grilled vegetables, or cover and store in an airtight container in the refrigerator for up to 5 days.

FOR THE VEGETABLES:

½ cup of oil (again, use a blend of 25 percent olive
   with 75 percent corn)

1 serrano chili cut into ⅛-inch-thick circles, seeds
   and all

1 teaspoon minced garlic

1 teaspoon salt

1 teaspoon black pepper

2 green zucchini, cut lengthwise into ¼-inch-thick
   slices (so that you have nice long strips that
   won't fall through the grill)

2 yellow squash, cut lengthwise into ¼-inch-thick
   slices

1 head fennel, cut lengthwise into ¼-inch-thick
   slices (leave the root on and discard after grilling)

2 chayote (Mexican squash), peeled, sliced into
   ¼-inch-thick slices, and seeded (or you can let
   the pit fall out when it's grilling)

4 to 6 cilantro sprigs

Corn tortillas, for serving

Pico de Gallo (recipe follows)

Crumbly Mexican cheese (optional—*queso cotija*
   would be a great match)

1. Preheat grill over medium–high heat. In a medium-size
bowl, combine the oil, serranos, garlic, salt, and pepper and
stir well. Lay your veggies on a sheet pan and, using a pastry
brush, coat each side with this chili–garlic–oil mixture. Flip
and brush the other side.

2. Grill until marked on both sides (and until the veggies
become tender), about 2 to 4 minutes per side. Slice the
grilled veggies horizontally into ⅛-inch-wide strips.

3. Heat comal or oven to 350° to warm the corn tortillas.

4. Heat the grilled vegetables in a pan with a little oil. Toss in the cilantro pesto, a little at a time, until you like the way it tastes.

5. Spoon the grilled vegetables tossed in cilantro pesto on top of the tortilla. Place 1 tablespoon of pico de gallo and some cilantro sprigs on top of the vegetables. Add cheese if desired.

Serve immediately.

PICO DE GALLO:

> 2 cups seeded tomatoes, cut into ¼-inch dice
> ¾ cup white (or Spanish) onion, cut into ¼-inch dice
> 2 or 3 serrano chilies, stemmed and diced, seeds
>   and all
> Juice of 2 fresh-squeezed limes
> 3 tablespoons chopped fresh cilantro
> 1 teaspoon salt, or to taste

1. Combine all of the ingredients in a medium-size bowl. Cover with plastic wrap and let sit at room temperature for an hour.

2. Taste again and adjust seasoning if necessary. Serve or store in an airtight container in the refrigerator for up to 4 days.

Adapted from Sue Torres.

Naomi Pomeroy's Creamy Asian Tomato Soup

This is a very fast and simple soup to make. The light coconut milk makes it creamy without being overly rich.

serves 4

- 2 tablespoons cooking oil
- 1¼ cup onion (chopped)
- 2 cloves garlic (1 rounded tablespoon)
- 1 28-ounce can chopped canned tomatoes
- 1 teaspoon kosher salt
- ½ teaspoon pepper
- ½ teaspoon paprika
- 1 tablespoon dark soy
- 2 teaspoons fish sauce
- 1 can low-fat coconut milk
- 1 tablespoon sugar
- 1 tablespoon red wine vinegar, or to taste
- ⅔ cup (or more) water to thin

1. Heat cooking oil in heavy-bottomed pot. Cook onions until translucent and add garlic. Cook for a minute more.

2. Add chopped tomatoes, salt, pepper, and paprika. Add soy, fish sauce, and then coconut milk. Simmer 5 minutes to meld flavors together. Add sugar and vinegar and adjust seasonings to taste.

3. Puree in a blender until completely smooth. Serve in bowls with optional garnish of chopped cilantro.

Adapted from Naomi Pomeroy.

Michelle Bernstein's Watermelon and Tomato Salad with Feta and Olives

"We're in the heat, so I crave cool/crispy/crunchy salad all the time," says Michelle Bernstein. "I love acid, particularly vinegar." This salad is typical of how Michelle likes to eat. Perfect for a summer dinner when you don't want to turn on the stove.

serves 6

4 cups (about ¼ of a medium watermelon) seedless watermelon or regular seeded watermelon, diced (½ inch)

2 large beefsteak tomatoes cut into 8 wedges each

2 cups peeled English (seedless hothouse) cucumbers, ¼-inch-thick diagonal slices

1 cup crumbled feta cheese, preferably French (about 4 ounces)

1 cup pitted Niçoise olives

2 tablespoons dill leaves

Red wine vinaigrette (recipe follows)

1. Put the watermelon, tomatoes, cucumber, feta, olives, and dill in a large bowl. Drizzle with half the vinaigrette and toss gently, taking care not to break up the fruit and vegetables. Add more dressing if desired and toss again.

2. This salad can be made the night before you serve it and refrigerated, but in that case, don't add the watermelon until ready to serve; refrigerate the watermelon separately. Let the salad and watermelon come to room temperature and toss together just before serving.

3. Divide among four to six salad plates and serve.

RED WINE VINAIGRETTE

You need barely any salt to make this dressing; the feta cheese and olives bring a lot to the dish.

>   2 tablespoons red wine vinegar
>   ¼ teaspoon garlic powder
>   ¼ teaspoon onion powder
>   ¼ teaspoon dried oregano
>   ¼ teaspoon za'atar (optional)
>   ½ cup olive oil
>   Kosher salt and freshly ground pepper to taste

Put the vinegar, garlic powder, onion powder, oregano, and za'atar in a small bowl. Whisk in the olive oil and season to taste with salt and pepper. The vinaigrette can be refrigerated in an airtight container for up to three days.

Adapted from *Cuisine à Latina* by Michelle Bernstein and Andrew
Friedman. Houghton Mifflin Harcourt, 2008.

BEHIND THE LESSONS:

Eric Ripert's Cookbooks

Tucked beneath the Midtown skyscraper that houses Le Bernardin is Eric Ripert's office. It's nothing fancy—employees, coffee, desks, papers, inside jokes. Then, in the conference room where we sit across from each other for an interview, there is a hidden trove: a floor-to-ceiling library of cookbooks. They are in French and English, and include encyclopedias of technique, titles by legends like Paul Bocuse and Ripert's mentor, Joël Robuchon, some recent editions by cutting-edge innovators such as David Chang and Grant Achatz, as well as home-cook classics of his adopted hometown, like Molly O'Neill's *New York Cookbook*. This impressive collection is just the overage from Ripert's home stash. "I have so many in my apartment, I had to bring them here," he says. "I still have too many."

Ripert has been Le Bernardin's executive chef since he was twenty-nine years old; within a year he won the understated but luxurious seafood restaurant a four-star rating from the *New York Times*, and later the maximum three stars from Michelin. He has wowed critics with dishes like a sampling of four fluke ceviches that, wrote the *Times*'s Frank Bruni in 2005, "turns into a world tour. First up . . . fish that has been marinated in lime, cilantro and onion: Peru. Next, olive oil, tomato and basil are thrown into the mix: the Mediterranean. After that comes the addition of ponzu: Japan. And then the fish is finished with a splash of coconut milk: Thailand."

Suffice to say, Ripert knows what he's doing without consulting cookbooks. He has no need to, for instance, check a dog-eared page on how to make hard-boiled eggs. (Add eggs to boiling water? Put them in cold water, then boil? Why can I never remember this?[1]) For Ripert, the books are much more than reference.

"I have collected cookbooks since I was fifteen years old. It's a way for me to daydream, escape, relax, and get inspired. I can travel without getting on a plane. For example, I can flip through a book on Indian home cooking and feel like I'm in someone's kitchen in Delhi. In the middle of winter I can daydream about summer in the South of France just by looking at a Mediterranean cookbook."

The books in the office sometimes serve a practical purpose: His sous chefs will browse the photos for ideas, or pick up a seasonal book to be reminded of what produce is coming up at the market. They will come downstairs to read and share new inspirations with the rest of the staff by jotting them down on a whiteboard. The library also speaks to Ripert's own curious mind. He has stayed at the top of his profession by, in part, continuing to learn, to explore.

"I have always had a passion for eating. From a young age I was in the kitchen with my mother and grandmothers, tasting every kind of food they prepared. There are very few things I do not like to eat. My whole life has been this way, and I think this curiosity and love of food helps keep my mind open to trying new ingredients that sometimes find their way on our menu." When Ripert and I met he had recently encountered fresh bergamot for the first

---

1 The answer is: Place eggs in cold, salted water; bring to a boil; lower heat to simmer for 5 to 8 minutes, then drain.

time—most people know it only as the perfumey element in Earl Grey tea. "I had never seen fresh bergamot," he says with wonder. "It's actually like a lemon. The juice is very sour, very acidic. That was the latest one."

He tries new things at home—even if they are new only to him. Though he rarely eats pasta, he tells me, "The other day I surprised myself by making a delicious lasagna. I was so happy with myself! Everybody was laughing: 'What's so amazing? You made *lasagna*? Big deal.' I don't know, but I'm so happy!'"

Novelty, exploration, transporting cookbooks—all these things contribute to Ripert's continuing love affair with the kitchen. "If I don't love it, I'm stopping immediately," he says. "But it's not even a question I ask myself. It's a passion. When you have a passion you don't question it. Do it and have pleasure in doing it."

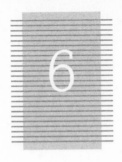

EAT IN OFTEN

I'M SITTING IN Tom Colicchio's office reading a menu upside down on his desk. On it is the lineup for that night's Tom Tuesday Dinner, a weekly private dining room experience at which the *Top Chef* head judge himself prepares a frequently changing tasting menu for about thirty-two people lucky enough to score a reservation (and with more than $200 to drop on a meal). This evening's diners will be treated to the following: butter-poached oyster; Jerusalem artichoke velouté; turbot with truffle butter; roasted lobster cacciucco (a seafood stew); Columbia River sturgeon; poached capon; black-truffle-stuffed porchetta; venison with mushrooms, lady apple, and honeyed turnips; grapefruit-Aperol sorbet; and a chocolate caramel tart.

Two nights earlier, Colicchio was cooking for an even more elite gathering: his family. On the menu? Pasta and broccoli, boiled in the same pot. This is shockingly close to how *I* make pasta and vegetables.

Cooking at home is (sorry, restaurant folk) better for you than eating out. It's cheaper, and you are unlikely to hide duck fat, sugar, or butter from yourself. "I don't go out as much these days, because I want to control what I eat," says Michelle Bernstein. "If I do go out, it's for food I don't know how to make, like sushi." Mark Bittman has noticed, "My caloric intake is probably double on the days I go out to dinner. You might have another course; the portions are bigger; you end up eating dessert; you have an extra glass or two of wine. At home, not so much."

Still, cooking for yourself or a family can be a challenge when it must be wedged in between work and sleep. I see the stress of home-cooking written on the faces of my coworkers. A meeting scheduled for five thirty can mean the difference between preparing a meal to be enjoyed on real plates, or coming home ravenous with enough energy only to order dinner over the phone. Cooking needs to be easy or you're apt to fall back on takeout or less healthy "convenience" foods. But it shouldn't be as easy as unwrapping a package and popping it into the microwave. Michael Psilakis knows from experience that eating better "involves, at some point, having to cook food."

I'm on board with that directive: I want to cook food. For me, the biggest obstacles are inertia, lack of preparation, and unresolved issues of timing, which I blame on having watched too many cooking scenes in movies, beginning with the bowl of spaghetti carbonara that Meryl Streep produces effortlessly during a sleepover date with Jack Nicholson in *Heartburn*. But as I proved to myself, they are not insurmountable. So, with the end goal to eat better and more healthfully, several chefs offered ways to eat at home more easily and affordably, drawn on their own experience in both their restaurant and home kitchens.

"Most of the meals I eat away from work are at home," says

Colicchio, whose New York City apartment kitchen isn't any bigger than my own. Before he was a dad of three, he used to go out to eat quite a bit. "Now, if I'm not at my own restaurant, one of the last places I want to be is at a restaurant." Several chefs felt the same way. Their chief complaint about staying in? They hate doing dishes. No one has figured out an acceptable solution to this yet.

Lesson 35: Smart chefs don't mistake home cooking for restaurant cooking

What do chefs eat at home? They have access to the best ingredients, and know how to do amazing things with them. "If people think we're home eating foie gras sandwiches, we're not," says Alex Guarnaschelli. "I make a lot of the food that I make on my cooking show." That includes homey American classics like roast chicken, green salads, pork chops with apples. Nothing that requires a blowtorch.

Says Sang Yoon, "My whole life has been spent in fine dining, so people think, 'You must scramble copious amounts of caviar into your eggs every day.' " Not so much, he assures me.

Yoon is an avowed bachelor ("I haven't bit on any of the five marriage ultimatums I've received," he tells me with a little laugh) whose home kitchen is stocked like a college kid's. Instant oatmeal. Soft tofu, which he heats and eats frequently, because he knows it is healthy and because it is an effective Sriracha delivery system. (Sriracha is that pepper sauce in the bottle with the rooster on it, ubiquitous in Vietnamese and Thai restaurants.)

"It's false to think that every single chef—save Alice Waters—on a day off, goes through the steps that they go through in their restaurants to prepare certain dishes," says Nancy Silverton. "We are very spoiled by having a brigade of prep cooks, dishwashers, and people to help us to create the layers of flavor that we do at our restaurants."

At home, you need to be your own prep cook. When you have time on a weekend, make some stock, a tomato sauce, or a versatile vinaigrette; precut your vegetables for tonight's dinner while you're waiting for your oatmeal to cook. She goes further: Not everything needs to be prepared from scratch. In fact, Silverton wrote a cookbook devoted entirely to cooking at home with familiar jarred, boxed, and canned ingredients. "There are a lot of things out there that are time-saving, or products from cans and jars and boxes that we use anyway, like anchovies, or capers. They have such concentrated flavors that they will add complexity to a dish."

To be sure, she's as concerned as anyone about avoiding additives like high-fructose corn syrup, preservatives, and MSG, and uses only products that don't contain them. This is not Nancy Silverton's take on *Semi-Homemade Cooking with Sandra Lee*; she makes a clear distinction between convenience products that fake a dish (like macaroni and cheese from powder in a box) and smart substitutions that simplify a dish (like a can of all-natural lentil soup in place of cooking lentils from scratch). She got the notion after reading an interview with Thomas Keller, in which he said he came home after work and often warmed up a can of Progresso lentil soup. Below, she shares a recipe in which she strains the soup to make a lentil base for quickly cooked salmon. Once the can is open, you can practically make it with one hand.

It's true that, like Silverton, Thomas Keller isn't a snob about store-bought shortcuts. The youngest of five boys raised in Palm Beach, Florida, by his mother, Betty, after their parents divorced, Keller grew up on eating things like chili dogs cooked by his older brothers while mom worked nights managing a continental restaurant. "You remember surf and turf? Fettuccine Alfredo? We didn't have specialized restaurants. Steak house and continental were the top-shelf restaurants," he recalls. These days, Keller could whip up his own ketchup without breaking a sweat. But he has often remarked that no gourmet or all-natural version pushes the same flavor button in most Americans, himself included, as an ordinary bottle of Heinz.

That's not an unimportant reason for turning to some time-tested staples—food memories are among our most indelible, and should be respected. Keller has recounted in detail a dinner he prepared in 2008 that he and his father enjoyed out on his porch. The centerpiece was one of Ed Keller's favorites: barbecue chicken, sauced from a bottle. The meal, rounded out by mashed potatoes, braised collard greens and strawberry shortcake, turned out to be his father's last; the senior Keller died at the age of eighty-six the following day. "It was a good dinner," Thomas writes in *Ad Hoc at Home*. "And now I am unspeakably grateful to have made it." He then shares all the recipes to re-create that dinner, gently instructing those of us who do to buy a bottled barbecue sauce "with some integrity, preferably from a small producer." I think about this instruction in particular when I'm cooking for my son. I would love if the flavors for which he is someday nostalgic come from foods with some integrity, and that will happen only if those are the products stocked in our pantry.

Lesson 36: They cook and eat simply at home

When I catch up with him, after meeting at Per Se, Keller tells me that he eats a lot of meals, dinner mainly, in his Napa Valley restaurants. He might have "family meal" with his staff before service, or once a week he'll go out to eat. But lunch, fit in around work and regular workouts, is most often put together in his white-cabineted Yountville home kitchen. What he makes for himself is easy, healthy, and, he allows, fairly repetitive. "I'll have a bowl of quinoa with some hummus, and I'll braise off some kale or broccoli—some vegetable—mixed together with some olive oil and vinegar. Sometimes I'll add a can of good Italian tuna fish. I eat that probably four to five times a week," he tells me. "If I'm feeling ambitious, I'll put a pot of beans on."

When he is home in the evening, he sometimes might have the same thing for dinner. The food for which he is known is almost surreally labor-intensive and relies on a sumptuous array of ingredients from caviar to venison to young ginger; the food that keeps his body humming is accessible, nearly vegetarian, and simple to throw together.

Another illustrious, high-wire chef, Laurent Gras, is best-known for the sophisticated seafood fare he created at Chicago's L2O. After earning three Michelin stars for the restaurant, he departed for New York with plans to open a less formal spot. At work his tools included tweezers for precision placement of delicate elements, and a Gastrovac, a $6,000 vacuum device that allows one food to take on the flavor of another through "cold impregnation." (The terminology comes from the Gastrovac catalog; I couldn't make it up.) At home it's another story. First off, he's happy to let his wife, Jennifer, do a lot of the cooking. But when he does cook for the two of them, you wouldn't mistake it for the food that made his reputation at L2O. "What I cook [at a restaurant] is really what I love. What I eat is for me to be healthy." As for his tools? Knives and pots and that's about it.

"If I want vegetables, I peel them, cut them, cook them, eat them. Simple," Gras explains, adding that he uses only olive oil to dress them, never butter, which I found surprising from a Frenchman who used pounds of melted butter at his restaurant as a poaching medium. What else? If he's in training on the bicycle—Gras is also a competitive distance cyclist—dinner might be pasta with vegetables, shellfish, or beef ragù. Otherwise, it's "fish baked with lemon juice, maybe rice, or a steak and a potato. Always a salad. Then we have fruits, yogurt." He doesn't bother much with spices, except maybe cayenne or black pepper and salt. Imagine the minimalist appeal of your refrigerator and pantry if this were the way you ate. Then imagine how good you would feel if this were the way you ate. Let your meals out be complicated; home can be a refuge of ease and good eating.

A few words about cooking from recipes. Chefs don't, really; they write them only because they need to give instructions to their restaurant crews or want to publish a cookbook. I love cookbooks, I read and use recipes, and it never occurred to me to not include them in this book. But I feel at my most competent and relaxed in the kitchen when I cook without one. If you're cooking simply, you may not need a recipe either.

Another way to lessen your reliance on recipes, says David Waltuck, of New York's storied Chanterelle restaurant, is to find a couple of dishes you like to eat, "and do them over and over and over again." From his perspective the most significant difference between home cooks and restaurant cooks is that the latter group prepares food over and over again, *all the time.* "So you learn, even if you're not brilliantly talented. You learn to put something in the pan, and wait a certain amount of time, and you smell, hear, look at it, and see when it's time to turn it."

Another reason to ditch recipes? "To write a recipe, you have to quantify everything," says Waltuck. "But everything is not quantifiable—it's what you like. There's not an exact amount, unless it's a baking thing, where there is chemistry. Use a little more garlic, or a little less garlic; it doesn't make any difference. Just *boom,* there's some garlic. *Boom,* it sizzles." Not having to measure an exact half tablespoon of a recipe's called-for uniformly minced garlic should free you up to cook more quickly, and hopefully more often. For his dinners, he says, "I just kind of improvise." After he made the career change from chef-owner of his own acclaimed restaurant to consulting for a restaurant group, he eats in quite often. "I'm busy during the day, and free at night. But by the time I get home there's not a lot of time to go shopping and cook. It's usually a sauté or some pasta. If I somehow have a moment, I'll make stock, but usually I don't. It's just that fifteen-minute dinner."

Lesson 37: Smart chefs don't mess up the whole kitchen

You probably don't even need a recipe for this, but here it is, courtesy of Chef Colicchio. Pasta and Broccoli in One Pot: "Boil the water, chop broccoli and garlic, throw in the pasta, throw in the broccoli and sliced garlic, drain it, put it back in the pot, add olive oil, lots of black pepper, Parmesan cheese, serve it. One pot. One of my favorite things to make at home."

Sang Yoon cooks at home rarely, but when he does he's also a big fan of the one-pot meal: soups, stews, casseroles, or curries. "In restaurants it takes so much equipment; at home I literally try to figure out what will take the least amount of effort and the fewest objects to wash, because I don't have my crew picking up after me. But I also think that one-pot meals are incredibly soul-satisfying, comforting."

Ever since his wife, Sandra, turned him on to this trick, Eric Ripert will cook fish or chicken in the toaster oven. "Amazing," says Ripert. "A piece of halibut in three minutes—you cannot mess it up!" Like any New Yorker, Ripert has friends with small apartments who use their real ovens for storage. So he's become a bit of an evangelist for toaster oven cooking, in life and on his Web site, AvecEric.com. (His recipe for Toaster-oven Chicken Paillard follows.)

Lesson 38: They get someone to cook for them

Perhaps you are reading this and thinking: *But I don't cook much!* Even if you are not the person in your home who handles the meals, it helps to think about the food that's coming in and how it's prepared. "To become interested in what you eat is the first step to healthy eating," says Masaharu Morimoto, who lost the forty pounds he put on due to absentmindedly ending his nights with big bowls of ramen. "Be knowledgeable about food ingredients," he advises. "Know which ones are low in calories and how to make those low-calorie foods tasty."

This doesn't mean you have to be the one to cook them.

Maybe a family member or a friend is willing to support your efforts to eat better. (I have loads of single pals who say they love to cook but won't do it for just themselves; is one of them your neighbor?) The first time I offered to make dinner for my husband (then boyfriend) in his apartment, he happily accepted, then said, "Oh, I suppose I'll have to call and have the gas to the oven turned on." In his refrigerator I found nothing but frozen lasagna, orange juice, and martini olives. He is really not a cook.

Morimoto, on the other hand, is certainly capable of preparing a meal for himself. But when cooking is how you make your living, it's nice to come home and have someone else take over kitchen patrol. If you are fortunate enough to have that be a person who cares deeply about your well-being, all the better. His wife, Keiko, favors traditional Japanese dishes that are light and full of vegetables like kinpira gobo (braised burdock root), and gomae (blanched spinach with sesame paste). When Morimoto decided to lose some weight, he stopped eating ramen. Instead, his wife buys shirataki noodles, which are made from konnyaku, a tuber that is very high in fiber and has virtually no calories. But they don't eat Japanese all the time. "She cooks shirataki pasta just like regular pasta—with fresh tomatoes, garlic, and basil—so you can still enjoy an Italian-style dish."

Morimoto says that having a pretty strict diet at home—one that is monitored by his wife—frees him up to eat as he likes elsewhere. "When I go out, I like trying out interesting food as a chef. This way, I care less about calories."

Lesson 39: Smart chefs keep the food they want to eat on hand

"I always eat pretty light," says Wolfgang Puck. "In our restaurant we don't really have heavy things sitting around. I eat a lot of fish. I love wild Alaskan salmon, which we get a lot here."

You may be tempted to say: "Well, if my kitchen were stocked like the one at Spago, I'd eat well too." But there's no reason not to keep your freezer and pantry full of the sorts of foods you love and that fit into the way you want to eat. I know that the nights when I'm seriously out of everything are when I end up eating Chinese takeout or pizza. Keep the food you want to eat around you.

"Have a terrific pantry," advises Lachlan Mackinnon-Patterson. "Buy great dry goods. One bottle of olive oil that you really love, one red wine vinegar you think is great." You will still have to do some shopping, but just for a couple of fresh items. "A head of Bibb lettuce, tossed with red wine vinegar and olive oil and a little salt and some chicken and you have a damn good salad that is fast and delicious and good for you."

When you have the opportunity, shop for the week ahead all at once. Over drinks at a book party, I asked David Waltuck about his most recent shopping trip, playing "what's in your basket?" with a renowned chef who cooks at home regularly. "We did a week of shopping at Fairway," he says of the famous New York emporium. "I bought a piece of beef fillet that I roasted; I don't love beef fillet, but it was cheap, so I bought it. I bought a lot of vegetables: broccoli, haricots verts, bok choy, tomatoes, and cheese." For dinner that night he unpacked pork cutlets, which "I pounded out, and did a version of saltimbocca: prosciutto, sage, marsala, a little chicken stock and butter."

One thing running a restaurant teaches you is that food that goes unused is money that is thrown out. You'll want to use it all, and to get it to stick around until you do. Marcus Samuelsson is a fan of repurposing leftovers. "Plan out the week and buy things that make three days of meals," he advises. "Roast chicken on Sunday, then chicken soup on Monday, and then a chicken pasta on Tuesday night." For this to work, you have to buy and cook enough food to yield true leftovers—the most likely thing to be tossed out is a sliver of, say, cooked salmon that is too small to make a meal for even one person. It will sit in your refrigerator as a tiny monument to a dinner you cooked until it turns on you and you have to get rid of it.

Jacques Torres, who says he tends to nibble late at night on whatever is hanging around from dinner, portions out his leftovers for future meals and puts them immediately into the freezer, so he isn't tempted to revisit them the same night. A tip about freezing leftover meats, from Mark McEwan: "With chicken, be careful not to overcook it, so it doesn't dry out" during freezing and reheating. "You can also vacuum-pack and freeze steaks if you buy good-quality meat that isn't too aged. Typically hormone-free products are not as aged."

McEwan also likes making a big portion of a flexible dish that tastes just as good a day or two after it's prepared. One of his favorites is lentils, "cooked tender so they don't break apart. Throw in a little feta, onions, a fresh herb, and a nice Italian vinaigrette. It's a universal side dish."

Lesson 40: They eat only treats they make themselves

Consider the potato chip. A good one can be amazing, a perfect sweater set of salt and grease. But when you're avoiding processed foods, empty calories, and generally foods that come in plastic packaging, potato chips are not something you eat too often. I hadn't had any in years, I think. Then I decided to make them at home. (Sliced thin on a mandoline, fried in canola oil, drained on paper towels, and sprinkled with sea salt—very easy.) They were better than any I remember.

Andrea Reusing tells me she likes the idea of "reclaiming foods that you think of as 'purchased' foods, and bringing them back into the kitchen." This includes what a lot of people might consider junk food, but that can be a fine indulgence when it comes from your stove instead of a vending machine. Her treats are French fries ("you can have a lot of fun eating French fries if you make them yourself") and homemade mayonnaise ("what's better on grilled fish or a French fry than that?"). She doesn't prepare French fries or mayonnaise every day. That's the point—these aren't foods that should be eaten every day. Making them should be a little bit of a production, and the payoff should be worth it. If you're going to eat fries or mayo or other treats only rarely, why not have them be phenomenal? Another plus? "When it's flavorful, you don't need as much," says Reusing of her mayo, which she makes with a stick blender.

I part ways with Reusing in one respect. She says, "I wouldn't make homemade mayonnaise just for myself, but I would if I were having even just two people over." I am the opposite: I don't yet trust my mayonnaise-making skills to attempt it when guests are expected. Instead, I'll try my hand at mayonnaise (which involves tossing out failures that look more like egg smoothies) when I'm alone.

Lesson 41: **They get the right balance on their plates**

How to decide what to put on a plate? When putting together a dinner for herself at home, Reusing goes for "a protein-centered meal, but not too much protein. I think a mistake a lot of people make is overproteining; four to five ounces is enough. I try to make a very flavorful sauce, and I don't worry about the fat in the sauce, because I'm not using that much."

Michelle Bernstein has a similar take: "I try to make the protein the third-largest item on the plate. Protein used to be number one. Now the vegetable is number one, a grain is number two, and protein is number three."

Susur Lee also eats more vegetables than meat. "If you are going to eat a lot of meat," he advises, "you should eat at least the same amount of vegetables."

Chefs also think of balance in terms of hitting a lot of different notes: soft/crisp, creamy/crunchy, rich/light. "A dish that is heavy with too much cream and fat and cheese is just a bad dish, even if it is palatable and rich," says Matt Lee. "It's missing all these other pleasure points, like color, vibrancy, freshness, and textural contrast—there's a million things a dish like that ignores." Adds Ted Lee: "There's a tendency in a lot of Southern restaurant cooking to go big and decadent. But if you've got a beautiful piece of pork belly and you're going to serve it with a butter-bean ragout, please don't put pork stock in that butter-bean treatment, because I've already got richness on my plate. Bring a sour element or some fire to it."

A typical Michael Symon home dinner will have some meat in it, but it will start with a salad of raw, shaved vegetables dressed in citrus juice or red wine vinegar and olive oil. "Because I cook with so much protein and animal fats, I'll always balance it with something crisp and acidic. To me the most tragic dish ever is meat loaf and mashed potatoes—soft on soft." Marcus Samuelsson put it another way: "Why does everything have to be soft? We have the best teeth in the world! We do! Some stuff should be chewy."

Though he occasionally puts together a meat-free meal, Symon can't help but come up with meat-veg pairings. Recently, he says, "I made some slow-roasted beets and a quinoa-almond salad with feta, which my wife said was delicious. I said, 'I know—it would be great with some duck breast on top of it!' She's like, 'Why can't you just enjoy this?' I don't know. I can't stop thinking about it with duck."

Lesson 42: **They eat roast chicken**

I briefly entertained the notion of titling this book *When They're Not Cooking for You, Chefs Are Home Roasting Chicken*. Because whether the chefs grew up in Jersey or Texas, it didn't matter. Whether they were raised by parents from France or Haiti, it didn't matter. Whether they made their reputation in Latin fusion or rustic Italian cuisine, it just didn't matter. Whenever I asked a chef what he or she likes to cook at home, almost invariably the first response was, "Roast chicken." Believe me when I tell you that I did not solicit roast chicken stories; they simply poured forth.

Ironically, the only person who didn't offer a roast-chicken-at-home story was Thomas Keller, whose recipe for same is among the most searched on the Internet. When I ask him about it, he reminds me that he eats it frequently as part of the staff meals at his restaurants, or when dining as a customer at Bouchon. He did have this piece of advice, however: Temper your chicken before roasting—that is, bring it up to room temperature, to ensure even cooking. Home cooks "just don't temper their food," he says. "They are afraid to take the chicken out of their refrigerator and leave it out for two and half hours—they think they're going to die. But at every great restaurant, that's exactly what we do."

You may already have a trusted roast chicken method. Enjoy your favorite in the knowledge that, if you make one on a Sunday night when most chefs take off, there's a good chance that you and, say, Tom Colicchio are enjoying the same dinner.

Here, thoughts on roast chicken from . . .

- Michelle Bernstein: "If you wanted to roast a simple chicken and then take the skin off to eat it—which I think is a *travesty*, but some people like to do that—I would throw the chicken into a brine, and that would be a combination of four gallons water, a half cup salt, a little bit of agave for sweetness, and then peppercorns, fennel seeds, celery seeds, lemon or orange zest, all my favorite stuff. Then you throw that whole chicken in there, and weigh it down with a couple small plates, and leave it [refrigerated] at least five hours, or put it in before you go to sleep, which I love to do. Then wash off the chicken; stuff it with a couple of lemons or oranges or herbs. Rub it with a little olive oil, roast it nice and low at three twenty-five, then go up to four hundred to get it golden. [It's done when the thickest part of the thigh reaches 165°F.] Then you've got the most delicious chicken. You don't need sauce. You can roast it on top of some chopped vegetables. Add some favorite grains, like Kamut or farro or Jerusalem artichoke pasta, with some toasted garlic, and some salad. It's the perfect meal."
- Melissa Perello: "I try to salt the chicken ahead of time, like a dry brine, season it really heavily, wrap it back up, and let it sit in the refrigerator. Roast the chicken, and I'll serve the whole Dutch oven

on the table, with a salad. I'm also a huge fan of Judy Rodgers's Zuni Café's roasted chicken dish with the bread salad. She takes all the schmaltz and chicken liquor, tosses the bread in it, and roasts the bread until it gets really nice and crispy. That's tossed with hearty greens, like frisée and chicory. So I always throw in chunks of bread, quartered Meyer lemons, and potatoes."

- Cat Cora: "I do a really great saffron-honey roasted chicken. Warm the honey up and blossom the saffron in a little water and add it to the honey, and you just glaze the chicken three-quarters of the way through cooking, so it doesn't burn. My wife taught me how to make fantastic fennel chicken—lots of ground fennel on it, and salt and pepper."

- Marc Murphy: "Simple roast chicken. Potatoes. Whole roasted shallots. Rosemary. What else do you need?"

- Tom Colicchio: "I don't do fussy. Roast chicken with vegetables."

- Nancy Silverton: "There's a Peruvian chicken place near my house, where they roast their chicken in front of a wood fire. I think it's fantastic. So if I come home from work and I'm starving, I can do something with that roast chicken."

So be as fancy—or not—as you want, with this chefs' staple.

Eric Ripert's Chicken Paillard
with Tomatoes, Fennel, and Olives

Though he is known for fish professionally, at home Ripert rarely makes it. This is an unexpected preparation, and a neat trick for making dinner without heating the oven. (If you don't have a toaster oven, you can use a conventional oven at the same temperature and time, though it will take a big oven longer to preheat.)

serves 2

> 2 skinless, boneless chicken breasts, butterflied
>   and lightly pounded flat
> 1 shallot, minced
> 1 clove garlic, minced
> ½ cup cherry tomatoes, cut in half
> 1 small fennel, sliced thin
> ¼ cup green olives, pitted and sliced
> 1 tablespoon capers
> 2 sprigs thyme
> 3 tablespoons olive oil
> ¼ cup torn basil leaves
> Fine sea salt and freshly ground pepper

1. Preheat toaster oven to 400°F.

2. Season the chicken breasts on both sides with salt and pepper. Place the chicken in a baking dish.

3. Combine in a mixing bowl the shallots, garlic, tomatoes, fennel, green olives, capers, and thyme leaves. Drizzle the olive oil over the vegetables and season to taste with salt and pepper.

4. Cover the chicken with the tomato, fennel, and olive mixture and add a little more olive oil over and around. Bake the chicken paillard for 10 to 15 minutes until cooked through. Sprinkle the basil over the chicken and serve immediately.

Adapted from *Avec Eric: A Culinary Journey with Eric Ripert*,
by Eric Ripert. JohnWiley & Sons, 2010.

—

Tom Colicchio's Sturgeon Wrapped in Prosciutto

I joined Tom during a walk-through of the Craft kitchen as some of his staff was starting to prep dinner. On the menu that night was this dish, which we agreed could be easily replicated at home. If sturgeon is unavailable, another sturdy white fish such as cod or black cod (also known as sablefish) can be used. Cooking time will vary based on the thickness of the fillet.

serves 4

> 4 7-ounce, 1½-inch-thick sturgeon fillets
> Kosher salt and freshly ground pepper to taste
> About ¼ pound prosciutto, thinly sliced
> 3 tablespoons peanut oil (or other vegetable oil)
> 3 tablespoons butter
> 2 sprigs thyme

1. Season each of the fillets with salt and pepper. Wrap two pieces of prosciutto, slightly overlapping, around the center of each fillet (the prosciutto will not cover the ends of fish).

2. Warm the oil in a large skillet over medium-high heat. Add the fillets to the pan and cook until the pans are once again hot, 1 minute or so. Reduce the heat to medium and cook the fillets until the first sides are crisp, about 1 minute. Turn the fillet over and cook the second sides until they too are lightly browned, 1 to 2 minutes.

3. Turn each fillet onto a third side. Add the butter and thyme to the pan. Cook, basting the fish with butter until the third sides are also caramelized, another 1½ minutes or so. Rotate the fish once more and cook the final sides, basting frequently. (Cooked for a total of 6 minutes, the fish will be a little translucent at the center—reduce the heat and cook the fish longer for more well-done.) Slice and serve.

Adapted from *Craft of Cooking* by Tom Colicchio. Clarkson Potter, 2003.

Nancy Silverton's Seared Salmon with Lentils and Salsa Rustica

Besides the convenience of canned lentil soup, this recipe utilizes basil paste, which can be found in small jars or tubes. It's basically basil whirred with oil. Salsa rustica has nothing to do with the tomato-based condiment most people think of as "salsa." In fact, it's an unexpectedly satisfying mix of hard-cooked eggs, mint, and almonds.

serves 4

FOR THE SALSA:

¼ cup whole raw almonds, with their skins on

3 tablespoons extra-virgin olive oil, plus more to toss with the almonds

Kosher salt

2 large eggs

3 tablespoons finely chopped fresh mint leaves

1 heaping tablespoon basil paste

FOR THE LENTILS:

1 cup extra-virgin olive oil

2 large garlic cloves, grated or minced (about 2 teaspoons)

Kosher salt

Two 15-ounce cans of lentils, or two 19-ounce cans of lentil soup, rinsed and drained (about 3 cups)

4 6-ounce salmon fillets, about 1½ inches thick (preferably wild king salmon)

Kosher salt

Freshly ground black pepper

¼ cup canola oil (or other neutral-flavored oil)

Lemon, for squeezing over the fish

Sea salt

1. Adjust the oven rack to the middle position and preheat to 325°. Spread the almonds on a baking sheet and toast them in the oven, shaking the pan occasionally for even toasting, for 15 to 20 minutes, until they are lightly browned and fragrant. Remove the almonds from the oven, drizzle them with olive oil, sprinkle with kosher salt, and toss to coat. Let them cool, then coarsely chop.

2. To hard-cook the eggs, place them in a medium saucepan with enough water to cover, salt the water generously, and bring to a boil over high heat. Reduce heat to low and simmer the eggs for about 5 to 8 minutes, until the yolks are cooked but bright yellow. (Nancy sometimes puts an extra "tester" egg in the pot.) While they are cooking, fill a large bowl with ice water. When the eggs are done, drain and plunge into ice water to prevent further cooking. When they are cool, peel the eggs and separate the whites and yolks.

3. To make the salsa: Coarsely chop the egg whites and yolks, separately. Place both in a medium bowl. Add the almonds, olive oil, mint, and basil paste and toss gently to combine. Add salt if necessary.

4. To make the lentils, heat ½ cup of the olive oil with the garlic and a pinch of salt in a medium saucepan over medium-high heat and sauté for about 90 seconds, until the garlic is soft and fragrant, stirring constantly so the garlic doesn't brown. Add the lentils and cook for about 3 minutes, stirring occasionally until they're warmed through. Remove the pan from the heat and season with salt to taste.

5. Rinse the salmon fillets under cool water and pat dry with paper towels, and season both sides with kosher salt and ground pepper.

6. Heat the canola oil in a large skillet over high heat for 2 to 3 minutes (you will be able to smell the oil, but it should not be smoking). Put the fillets in the pan, skin-side down. Place a flat lid or plate smaller than the diameter of the pan on top of the fish and press down gently for about 4 minutes (this helps render a crispy skin). Remove the lid or plate and reduce the heat to medium. Slide a thin spatula under the salmon to release any sticking spots and turn them on their sides; cook for 1 minute on each of the two sides. Turn and cook the salmon on the fourth side for 1 minute. Turn off the heat and let the salmon cook from the residual heat of the pan for 1 minute more.

7. Spoon the lentils onto four plates, evenly, and place the salmon skin-side up on top of the lentils. Squeeze a few drops of lemon juice and sprinkle sea salt over each fillet. Spoon the salsa rustica on top.

Adapted from *A Twist of the Wrist: Quick Flavorful Meals with Ingredients from Jars, Cans, Bags, and Boxes* by Nancy Silverton. Knopf, 2007.

BEHIND THE LESSONS:

Nate Appleman's Career Change

For a few months in 2010 food bloggers and the generally curious were stopping by the Chelsea location of the Chipotle Mexican casual chain to confirm for themselves: Was a past winner of a James Beard Rising Star Chef award and *Food & Wine* Best New Chef really slinging shredded beef and tortillas? He was.

Nate Appleman's unusual path began with a formal education at the Culinary Institute of America, followed by travels through Italy, where he learned to butcher meat and cure his own *salumi*, and became one of the few Americans recognized as an authentic pizzaiolo. (Italians don't mess around with their pizza chefs; they give certificates and everything.) Later, in San Francisco, Appleman was the chef at two acclaimed Italian restaurants, SPQR and A16. Devastated Bay Area foodies declared it "Nateaggedon" when he left for New York in 2009 to be a chef-partner at the downtown upscale pizzeria Pulino's, where he hushed critics with goat meatballs, and fed scenesters with burgers available only after midnight. But even with his success, he soon lobbed another curveball: He left Pulino's and reemerged behind the counter at a Chipotle. The response in the blogosphere was a collective "Wha . . . ?"

Why did he do it? "I realized I'd lost touch with what I loved about cooking. Being a chef now, you expedite tickets all night long. My life's ambition is not ripping tickets off a machine and reading them to cooks. You know, it's actually cooking and training people," says Nate. "I realized I like to develop people; that's the best aspect of what I do."

While he can be found behind the counter, he isn't a typical counter worker, of course. He's a culinary manager, developing recipes that will be used by the restaurants nationwide, and figuring out how to bring his nose-to-tail cooking to a chain of that size. "My mission is to use the whole animal." The day I visited him in his development kitchen, we did a chorizo tasting together: seven variations on pork and chicken sausage blends. With another company chef, we debated using skin ("it adds an unctuous quality"), fresh oregano, more vinegar or less. (When they said one sample "eats really well," I realized that, among other things, what distinguishes me from a professional chef is the comfortable use of "eat" as an intransitive verb.)

It is a fairly limited menu: tacos, burritos, salads. But if anyone suspected that he had checked his creativity at the door, Appleman reemerged publicly to compete for charity on *Chopped All-Stars*, and—with a crazy dish of honey and grapefruit semifreddo with chickpea-and-sesame caramel and a chayote salad—won the top prize of $50,000 for the Kawasaki Disease Foundation. It was a personal victory as his son, Oliver, had been diagnosed with the syndrome, which caused him heart problems. Oliver is doing well today, and Appleman points to another benefit of his new gig: most nights off.

Asked whether there is anything he misses about fine dining, he thinks for a few moments and then can come up with only one: He liked it when other chefs came to his restaurant and he could cook for them. "I still see them, but Daniel [Boulud] is not coming into Chipotle."

Stranger things have happened.

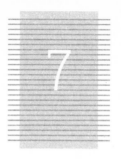

EAT YOUR
VEGETABLES

"THERE ARE PICTURES of me all over the Internet with a pig slung over my shoulder," says Naomi Pomeroy, the self-taught chef-owner and sometime butcher of Portland's Beast, a restaurant known for homey fare that she calls "refined French grandmother." When the picture appeared in a magazine article in which Pomeroy jokingly described herself and her sous chef as "two young, attractive ladies taking down some hogs," the backlash was immediate. "They slammed me for that, and for being a carnivore generally. What upset me is, I am one of the more vegan proponents out there. I don't feel great when I eat that much meat; I'm happy to admit that."

She can understand the confusion. "When you come to Beast you get the foie gras bonbon, and you get six decadent courses, a cheese course, a dessert course. But we don't eat that at all," says Pomeroy of herself and her almost all-female staff. "For lunch a couple of times a week I'll make a big batch of quinoa, and we eat vegan." In part this is because, she allows, "we all want to lose our ten or fifteen pounds."

This chapter tackles two ideas: eating less meat, and eating more vegetables. One involves a commitment to eat fewer animal products—a good idea for all the health reasons I'm sure you've heard before: less risk of cancer and heart disease, and other benefits bound to make your life longer and generally more pleasant. The second involves not merely replacing meat with cheese pizza and sesame noodles, but actually filling your meals with vegetables. Happily, making vegetables taste good with little effort is something chefs know about.

Lesson 43: Smart chefs have given a no-meat diet a chance

Spending time as a vegetarian will inform how you eat as an omnivore; chefs who have done so appear more conscious and conscientious about how they eat and how they live away from the kitchen or dining table.

Pomeroy is one of several chefs who surprised me with a vegetarian past. She was meat-free for seven years, starting with her senior year in high school, when she was suddenly turned off by the sound of her mother cutting up a chicken. She went back only when she became a personal chef and needed to taste the meat she was cooking for clients. At her own restaurant, she makes thoughtful choices about meat that perhaps only a former vegetarian would. She knows the farmers and how the meat she buys is raised. And because Beast serves just a fixed menu, when she butchers a pig she can use all the parts, a more ecologically and ethically sound use of the animal than catering to à la carte diners who order only pork chops.

Tom Colicchio, who went on to open Craftsteak, among other restaurants, was also a young vegetarian: "For a year, when I was twenty-two or twenty-three," he recalls. "I was in a restaurant and looked into a stockpot after the stock had been strained out of it, and it was just bones in there and it looked so disgusting. I said, 'I can't eat meat.'" That change led to others: He quit smoking, started running more. For that year, although he continued to work with meat, he didn't eat it. "It wasn't difficult; we're around more vegetables than we are meat or fish."

Gregory Gourdet, chef at Departure in Portland, Oregon, having been raised on a typically American omnivorous diet by his Haitian parents in Queens, went meat-free when he left home for school in Montana, having decided to become a wildlife biologist. In Missoula, his roommate "was a kid from Long Island who would cook all the time—that got me going." Two things subsequently happened: "One, I realized I wasn't as outdoorsy as I thought I was. Two, I realized I wanted to be a chef." While in college, he says, "I thought about how I perceived meat, and I was vegetarian for all four years." He eventually moved back to New York and, "as I segued into culinary school, I started eating fish and then I was full-on omnivore."

During the years that he was coming up in Jean-Georges Vongerichten's Manhattan restaurants, "I lived the fast chef life—I had plenty of *Kitchen Confidential* moments," he says, referring to the Anthony Bourdain bad-boy memoir. Gourdet and his pals "would cook all day, drink and stay out all night. We did lots of drugs and went to all the newest restaurants, bars, and clubs. Some nights we'd start off with croque monsieurs at Pastis. Maybe we'd be at Blue Ribbon getting the fried chicken and bone marrow or, if it was really, really late, at Cafeteria eating bacon blue cheese burgers and mac-and-four-cheese. Cigarettes too, of course. Needless to say I could only do this for so long before I realized something had to give. I jumped at the offer to move to California and do something different."

Everything was different: He dedicated himself to improving his health. No more cigarettes or drugs. "Everyone in California works out—more so than in New York. I joined the gym and went health nut: I started cutting out red meat and dairy and I started running more. I lost twenty pounds."

Today he says, "I don't enjoy the taste of red meat, and I don't miss cheese. I've been eating lighter foods for so long, whenever I eat something fried or creamy, I get the greasy mouthfeel. I don't like it." That said, he will cook you Asian-spiced pork belly at Departure, and he isn't averse to tasting at work.

I understand that contradiction. I was a vegetarian for twenty years. A few weeks after I started covering chefs as a journalist, I went to a promotional wine luncheon at Per Se, where each course was carefully paired with the client's wine. After some deliberation, I figured I'd just go with whatever was on the menu, whether fish, fowl, or fauna. It was Per Se, for goodness' sake. I was glad I did. When I saw another writer ask for steamed vegetables in place of the duck, I realized how ridiculous I was going to look navigating the food world with this self-imposed limitation. The duck—and the wine—convinced me I had done the right thing.

Today I still eat meat sparingly, with the awareness of someone who has made a choice to do so, and I am picky to the point of obnoxious about finding out from whence the meat on my plate has come. It is possible, I believe, to have the heart of a vegetarian and the palate of an omnivore.

Although Gourdet is no longer a hard-core veggie, the influence of that period still resides in how he cooks and eats. He trains hard as a marathoner, and says, "Throughout my day I'll have lean protein: eggs, chicken, turkey, nut and seed butters. I consume all the fruits and vegetables that I want—I don't limit those by any means. I drink fruit juice and use almond milk for my cereal or smoothies." Eating that way, he says, "I got extremely lean, and achieved a lot of fitness goals."

Lesson 44: Mark Bittman's vegan vampirism

If you're deciding to eat fewer animal products—dairy and eggs included—it can be helpful to give yourself some rules, so you're not dithering over every choice at every meal. Mark Bittman devised an easy strategy: He is vegan during daylight hours.

What *The Joy of Cooking* was to my childhood, Mark Bittman's *How to Cook Everything* will be for my son's. The big red book looms large in our kitchen. The first time I met Bittman was at a starry party for the launch of a public television series he appeared in, *Spain . . . On the Road Again*. Gwyneth Paltrow was there. Bono too. It was at the Spanish consulate in New York, and it was crowded and hot and people were pink-cheeked from the proximity to fame and possibly the prosecco. But even with all the A-listers in the room, I wanted to talk to Bittman about how he ate.

I caught up with him later at his office at *The New York Times*. He had lost a fair amount of weight, and was about to publish his book about "conscious eating," *Food Matters*. In it he delivers a persuasive argument for eating less meat and more plants that includes benefits not only for your health, but also for your wallet and for the health of the planet. But here, I'm concerned only with how the shift to part-time vegetarianism affected Bittman's waistline.

A few years back, when he was about thirty pounds over-weight, Bittman ran into some health troubles: His cholesterol and blood sugar were high and he suffered from sleep apnea. Where a more conventional doctor might have put him on Lipitor or other drugs, Bittman's doctor, whom he describes as an iconoclast, told him simply to give up eating any animal products—become a vegan.

"Did he know what you do for a living?" I ask. Besides writing cookbooks, for thirteen years Bittman developed recipes for his weekly "Minimalist" column in the *Times*.

"Of course, we've known each other for thirty years. He said, 'You're smart; figure something out.'"

Here's what he came up with: From the time he woke until the time the sun went down he wouldn't eat meat, dairy, eggs, sugar, pasta, or refined carbohydrates of any kind. At dinner, he would eat whatever he pleased, including any or all of the above. This might be a short leap for someone raised on grains and beans and tofu. But as a boy, Bittman was a New York street food gourmand. "I could eat seven hot dogs or four slices of pizza; I'm not exaggerating. Every chance I got I was out eating a knish or a corned beef sandwich."

After a month of this ritual of daytime veganism, he had lost fifteen pounds, without exercising at all. (Bittman isn't against exercise; at that point he had just had knee surgery. Eventually he returned to walking, biking, and then running.) "Fifteen pounds—pretty interesting," he remembers thinking. "Then I had my blood work done, and all the numbers were where they should be. Pretty interesting. So I kept eating that way. I lost another fifteen pounds and the apnea went away. Now I'm quite sure if I ate the way I used to I'd gain twenty pounds immediately."

Lesson 45: They see meat in the big picture—eating a lot is bad for not just you

When Nate Appleman resolved to lose weight, he found that sugar was easy to eliminate. Meat not so much. He describes himself as "a very meat person." But well into his career, he decided to eat less of it—and to fill more of his plate with vegetables. "There's no question that Americans consume more meat than they need," says Appleman. "And it's usually bad meat." By "bad" he means raised poorly: in inhumane factory farms, full of antibiotics and growth hormones. His way of cutting back on the quantity of meat he consumes is to focus on the quality. If you eat only good meat—grass-fed, hormone- and antibiotic-free, sustainably and humanely raised—you are going to eat less automatically, because it just isn't available at every restaurant you might frequent. "I'm wary of where I eat meat, and what kind of meat I'm eating," says Appleman. "I don't think it's a weight thing. I don't even know if it's a health thing," he says. "I think it's more like a moral thing."

Conversations with your server about meat sourcing may be awkward at first—I've gotten the long sigh from waiters as they trot back to the kitchen to ask whether the chicken is antibiotic-free—but worth it in determining whether you're sitting down to a meal that should include meat.

Lesson 46: They invite vegetables home . . . and don't let them exit through the garbage can

Confession: I'm excellent at buying produce; I'm somewhat less great at using what I've bought before it goes limp and brown.

I am always overly ambitious at the market, and then horribly regretful when sacrificing bendable carrots to the kitchen trash bin or discovering a cucumber, white with fuzz, at the back of the fridge.

"I think that's normal. You share that problem with millions of other people," Marcus Samuelsson tells me when I admit my produce neglect to him. His suggestion: Learn a couple of recipes that halt the decline of fresh fruits and vegetables. Rather than temper my enthusiasm at the green market, he advises, "Buy more! Make jam. Make a ketchup with jalapeño or raspberries." This is a twofold winner: You'll save your tomatoes but also reward yourself with beautiful homemade condiments, the better to dress fast meals of quickly cooked grains, fish or chicken, and vegetables.

There are, however, plenty of times you don't feel like sterilizing jars for jam. In fact, that describes most weeks in my house. As an alternative, I've become a fan of freezing fruit that I can tell isn't going to make it to Tuesday. Slice up a peach at its peak of ripeness, arrange the wedges on a plate so they aren't touching, and stick it in the freezer. When they're frozen, put them in a Ziploc bag. When you dig them out during winter, you will thank your thoughtful summer self.

It's also a good idea to add to your repertoire a few ways of coping with vegetables on the verge of being of interest only to historians. Alex Stratta opened my eyes to the pleasure of roasted lettuce. "If your romaine lettuce is starting to wilt, don't throw it away; cut it in half, dress it with olive oil, garlic, a little salt, and roast it. I love roasted lettuces," he says. Since trying that method, I've also taken to sautéing lettuce as if it were spinach, and each time I do I think back on the years when I believed that lettuce had to be crispy to be enjoyed. There is almost no vegetable that cannot become soup, along with an onion sautéed in some olive oil, and water or stock. Or when I have berries or fruit that appear to be going over to the dark side, I stew them quickly for a topping that enlivens oatmeal or pancakes or, when cooled, plain yogurt.

Even before you let produce get to the salvage point, it's better just to use what you've got. You don't need loads of recipes. Nate Appleman recalls a stew he made with his son by cleaning out the produce bin. "I just took all the vegetables that were in the fridge—I think there was some tomato, onions, which I sautéed, there was bok choy, carrots, and chickpeas. Then I made an egg-and-corn pancake—what else did I put in it?" He tries to remember. "Oh, sweet potato. It was sweet potato, egg, corn, and the greens from the bok choy." Not a conventional combination, but he believes that "as long as you use good ingredients, and you know how to use salt, you can make something really tasty without even trying. I literally take all the vegetables at home, throw them together, cook them, season them—I've used cumin, just to spice it up a little—and that's typically how dinner will go down." Another night it was "cauliflower, onion, pepper, and tomatoes, just jumbled. We got some mozzarella from a local place over in the East Village. I put some sesame seeds on it, and then we had avocado toast. That was our dinner."

That kind of improvisation is helped greatly by the CSA delivery Appleman gets regularly. A CSA (community supported agriculture) membership—sort of like a magazine subscription for local farm produce—is an easy way to get vegetables into your home, which, while it sounds obvious, is the first step to actually bringing them into your diet. "It's a way for farmers to 'clean their fridge,'" says Appleman. Andrea Reusing is a CSA member; so is Tom Colicchio. "We get a delivery of organic vegetables every week. So whatever shows up, I cook with," says Colicchio. Think of it as your own personal *Top Chef* challenge: What will you do with all that zucchini? How about those yellow beets? (He has a suggestion, below.)

Lesson 47: **They eat vegetables "nose to tail"**

Using every bit of the animal is justly popular today: Meat is expensive, waste is appalling, and there are some interesting and traditional preparations for the parts most of us rarely consider. But what about produce?

Many chefs are proponents of "nose to tail" vegetable use. For a while, Thomas Keller's California broccoli supplier was harvesting only the tops. "They were leaving the stems in the field, and I said, 'I want to buy those from you.' Because the stems, to me, are amazing," says Keller. "Peeled and blanched, they are just great. Asparagus stems, same thing. Artichokes actually have a long stem," he says, adding that they are usually removed, leaving only the globe for us to buy. When you can find the stems intact, "peel them down and you get that good center. And we do a lot with the ribs from the Swiss chard." (The very night I was writing these words I peeked online at the evening's menu at Per Se, which included a salad of caramelized sugar pie pumpkin, black winter truffle coulis, Cape Cod cranberries, Swiss chard ribs and pumpkin seed "aigre-doux." Don't the stems of chard leaves sound appealing in that lineup? (Aigre-doux is French for sweet-and-sour, by the way.) Says Keller: "We always try to use the entire vegetable."

I'm sure I threw out a small forest of broccoli stems before I learned that, liberated from their outermost husk, the stalks taste like a whole other vegetable, with the snap of celery, and less of broccoli florets' crucifer scent. Now I will use them in a stir-fry or chopped raw into salad. Scraps like the peelings, tops, and stems of vegetables are valued by chefs as a worthy addition to stock. And carrot tops—when I buy a bunch of carrots at the supermarket, I'm still asked whether I want the tops off. (As if removing a bouquet of carrot leaves is somehow going to make my load lighter on the walk home?) No, I don't want the tops off. If they are fresh and vibrant, they are great sautéed like any other delicate green, or used in a pesto variation.

Lesson 48: Smart chefs don't over-romanticize local and seasonal produce

What was interesting to me was that, while chefs are big fans of farmers' markets, they aren't all hung up on local and seasonal produce. Appleman remembers during his apprenticeship in Italy, "One of the guys I worked with, his family had a farm outside of the city and they ate that way. He said, 'We just had celery for three weeks. That's all we had. Braised celery, fried celery, celery salad.'"

Most of us crave more variety than that. In cold-weather climes, eating locally in winter is especially tough (you'd better love cabbage and potatoes). "I'm a big supporter of local, but the season is very short," says Mark McEwan of Toronto. "We stay with it when we can, but you can't eat squash the entire winter—that would get mundane. I'm not opposed to hot-house tomatoes from southern Ontario in the winter when they are organic." So if you can get a wider and more compelling variety at your supermarket, go for it. Don't let poor seasonal selection stop you from eating your vegetables.

Lesson 49: Smart chefs aren't vegetarian vegetable purists

Finally, if the way to get the vegetables out of the drawer and onto your plate is to serve them seasoned with something from the dairy or butcher's counter, a lot of chefs are completely with you on that. Scientists too: Several vitamins in vegetables are fat-soluble, and need that pairing to get absorbed. "A smoked turkey wing in collard greens makes them delicious," observes Andrea Reusing. "That, and not being afraid of putting a little butter and salt on string beans—kids will always eat them that way. *I* will always eat them that way. That balance works."

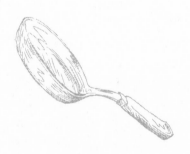

Tom Colicchio's Raw Yellow Beet Sandwiches with Avocado, Grapefruit, and Radish Sprouts

makes 4 sandwiches

2 medium yellow beets, peeled and julienned

1 tablespoon plus a drizzle of extra-virgin olive oil

Juice from half a lemon

1 teaspoon kosher salt, plus extra for seasoning

Freshly ground black pepper

1 large grapefruit

1 ripe avocado, halved, pitted, peeled, and thinly
sliced

8 slices Pullman bread, crusts removed

1 cup loosely packed radish sprouts

1. In a bowl, toss the beets in 1 tablespoon of the oil, lemon juice, 1 teaspoon of salt, and pepper to taste and set aside. Cut the grapefruit into supremes.★

2. Evenly layer the avocado slices on 4 slices of the bread. Drizzle some oil on the avocado and season with salt and pepper. Top with the grapefruit, yellow beets, and radish sprouts. Place the remaining 4 slices on top, cut into halves, and serve.

Adapted from *'wichcraft: Craft a Sandwich into a Meal—And a Meal into a Sandwich* by Tom Colicchio with Sisha Ortúzar. Clarkson Potter, 2009.

★ Making supremes of citrus sounds worrisome, but actually falls into the category of If I Can Do It, You Can Do It: Cut off the top (where the stem was) and bottom of a grapefruit or orange; then, with your knife following the curve of the fruit, cut off the peel and pith (the white layer) from the sides. Now, with the citrus segments exposed, cut each one away from the membrane so it slips out, holding its shape. If you've never done this before now, you should now recognize these pith-free segments from salads you've had in restaurants and should feel a deep sense of self-satisfaction at having duplicated them on your first try.

Mark Bittman's More-vegetable-than-egg Frittata

In this dish the vegetables, which vary to your taste, are "dominant and delicious," says Bittman, who recommends this frittata for brunch, dinner—anytime. Leave out the cheese for a lighter dish, or add a little chopped bacon, ham, or shrimp if you're otherwise inclined.

serves 2 as a main dish or 4 as a side

- 2 tablespoons olive oil or butter
- ½ onion, sliced (optional)
- Salt and ground black pepper
- 4 to 6 cups of any chopped or sliced raw or barely cooked vegetables
- ¼ cup fresh basil or parsley leaves, or 1 teaspoon chopped fresh tarragon or mint leaves, or any other herb
- 2 or 3 eggs
- ½ cup freshly grated Parmesan cheese (optional)

1. Put olive oil or butter in a skillet (preferably nonstick or well-seasoned cast iron) and turn heat to medium. When fat is hot, add onion, if using, and cook, sprinkling with salt and pepper, until it is soft, 3 to 5 minutes. Add vegetables, raise heat and cook, stirring occasionally, until they soften, from a couple of minutes for greens to 15 minutes for sliced potatoes. Adjust heat so vegetables brown a little without scorching. (With precooked vegetables, just add them to onions and stir before proceeding.)

2. When vegetables are nearly done, turn heat to low and add herbs. Cook, stirring occasionally, until vegetables are tender.

3. Meanwhile, beat eggs with some salt and pepper, along with cheese if you are using it. Pour over vegetables, distributing them evenly. Cook, undisturbed, until eggs are barely set, 10 minutes or so; run pan under broiler for a minute or two if top does not set. Cut into wedges and serve hot, warm, or at room temperature.

Adapted from *Food Matters: A Guide to Conscious Eating* by Mark Bittman. Simon & Schuster, 2009.

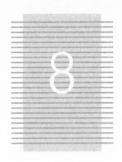

EAT OUT SMART

WHEN CHEFS GO out to restaurants, do they like to eat the way they cook? Or is a fancy restaurant meal more busman's holiday than relaxing treat?

Eating out, says Alex Guarnaschelli, "is important to recharge my own batteries. I love it when a chef comes into where I work. It's very flattering. 'Hey, I know what kind of schedule you have, and you took the time to come here and taste my food? Thanks!'"

But how do chefs eat when they go out to eat? Not necessarily the way they encourage customers to. Laurent Gras, who used to preside over a famed twelve-course tasting menu at L2O, never goes out for a big production like that. "I prefer to eat a three-course meal," says Gras. "I don't want to sit at the table for three or four hours. I like a more casual place, to meet friends, have a good time. When you work six days a week, eighteen hours a day, it's enough of the food world. You want something else."

Chefs realize there are times when their customers are like that too. They see a difference in how we order when we come in on Tuesday versus on Saturday. ("I can tell when someone has spent the whole week eating Lean Cuisine," notes one.) Yet chefs admit that while they don't want us to leave feeling too full and cursing them the next day, they do like it when we order a lot of food and booze—even if they themselves are famously fit.

"People will come in and say, 'I read that you're a cyclist and this healthy chef, and that's so great!' But that's not what we do here," says Quinn Hatfield of his eponymous French-inspired L.A. restaurant. "I'm capable of feeding myself the way I need to. Sitting down in front of a bowl of brown rice, I think of it as fuel. But that's not great dining."

Lesson 50: Smart chefs have an app for that

So if chefs won't play the role of health police for us, what's a diner to do? It is not a bad idea to remember that a menu is a listing of what is available; it isn't an instruction manual. Yet sometimes diners treat it like a guide to how a meal should be eaten. When Melissa Perello put a selection of small bites called bouchées at the top of her menu at Frances, she expected them to be ordered with a glass of wine at the bar, not as part of a meal. She soon found, however, that customers seated for dinner began treating them as a "pre-appetizer," and would routinely order four courses: a bouchée, an appetizer, an entrée, and dessert. They were eating more because more appeared to be on offer. More even than she had expected customers to eat. There's something about a hip restaurant that can make you feel like you should just go with the program. Well, don't.

Chefs themselves pay little attention to the implied suggestions of a menu. Quite often, they make meals of only appetizers. When I meet Donatella Arpaia for lunch, she orders a tomato salad and an appetizer of shrimp, mussels, and couscous. "If that's the only portion in front of me, I'm satisfied," she tells me. "If this were double the portion," she adds, tapping her second plate, "I'd eat double. I know myself. I know I can't control it if it's in front of me, so don't put it in front of me."

Besides offering more appropriate portions, "Appetizers are usually more interesting than entrees," says Tom Colicchio. Depending on the size, "I usually order three."

Lesson 51: They think about portion size

Chefs are customers as well as providers, so they consider this question from both sides of the plate. Colicchio's distaste for being served a too-big portion when he goes out influenced him when he was designing a menu for the restaurant he launched in 2010, Colicchio & Sons. "I made the portions purposely small. But because we serve expensive ingredients, and still have to charge a good amount of money for them, I got ripped apart. People complained, 'These portions are so small!' But if you eat an appetizer, entrée, and dessert, I can't believe you're not full." Nonetheless, he took the hint and made the portions slightly bigger. "People may skip dessert, but they want large portions," he noticed. "Then they won't eat the large portion."

I wonder why this is. Is it a problem stemming from the same root as the inflation of clothing sizes at the mall (what once was a ten is now an eight and so on)? Do diners feel somehow more virtuous if they can leave something behind on their plate, despite actually consuming a lot of food? Do we need a portion so big that we can sate ourselves and still appear to those across the table as if we are too dainty to finish an entrée?

Colicchio isn't sure either, though he perceives this as a uniquely modern American paradox. "Customers want to see that big portion, but then they get full or bored with it. It's the complete opposite of people who grew up during the Depression, or people in Europe during the war who ate everything on their plate because food was so scarce. In Europe, when I worked there, the chef always wanted to see the plates when they came back, and if they weren't finished, that meant something was wrong with the dish. Over there, you never heard, 'I'm just full.'"

Even chefs who are sensitive to this problem are probably serving too much food, because customers demand it. So when they eat out, they know that they likely won't be eating the whole thing; they can see when a portion is too big. It's worth taking the time to learn what a reasonable portion size—six to eight ounces of protein, about half a cup of pasta—looks like on a plate. Then you will be able to eat small portions of virtually everything you love.

For a variety of reasons, you won't be able to convince the waiter or the chef to serve portions of that reduced size. So take the advice of Ming Tsai: "The best thing to do is don't finish the plate. When you stop being hungry, stop eating."

Rick Bayless concurs on this point. He frequently orders both an appetizer and an entrée when he goes out with his wife and restaurant partner, Deann, and he loves sweets. On the job, he enjoys major multicourse "research" meals when he's traveling in Mexico for his PBS show. How does all of this not add up to obesity? It's an equation that can confound newer members of his TV crew.

"We just came back from a scouting trip," Bayless tells me when I meet him in Miami. "We have a new producer, and she said, 'Oh, my God, I'm going to gain ten pounds!' The rest of us said, 'What are you talking about? We eat like this every day! But we know when to stop.' Do I eat everything put in front of me? No. I know what my metabolism is."

This is where it may get tricky for those less experienced at eating this way: People who muddle through the week on watery "light" yogurt and plain grilled chicken are more apt to lose control when they treat themselves to a delicious meal on the weekend. You could maintain your weight that way, but it isn't much fun. In fact, it makes most days feel like penance for those few splurges.

Nate Appleman also finds limiting how much you eat more useful than trying to change the kinds of foods you eat. "We are creatures of habit—we're going to eat what we want. So portion control was a more practical way for me. For me, four ounces of meat is plenty."

If you find it too difficult to stop eating all that's on your plate, one answer is to order less, perhaps one meal between two people. "My wife and I will share a pizza and salad or split a bowl of pasta," says Mark McEwan. "We're generally eating half of what many people around us are eating." As a restaurateur whose profit depends on big tabs, isn't he bothered by people going halvsies? "No, I encourage it. It's nice to order family style in a restaurant, order plates to share, put your elbows on the table and relax."

Besides making the meal more interesting, sharing makes it more intimate. The first time I was introduced to Andrea Reusing, she was visiting New York and we met for lunch near Union Square. We might have hit it off anyway, talking about our kids and our shared foam-food fatigue (are aerosol carrots really necessary in this life?). But dipping your spoons into the same bowl of lemongrass-mussel soup is a fine way to make fast friends.

Another possibility is choosing a set menu at a restaurant where you trust the portions are likely to be appropriate. At Le Bernardin, for instance, "It's hard to overdo it with the portion we give you," says Eric Ripert, the chef there. "It's pretty calculated. The idea is to be at the end of your dinner neither hungry nor too full. We try to find the balance." There, diners get a prix fixe fish-based meal. "At lunch an appetizer is two to three ounces, and the entree is about eight ounces of protein. At night we have two appetizers, one cold, one hot, so the main course is six ounces," Ripert explains. He acknowledges that "if you were eating at Le Bernardin every night—with wine, bread, and dessert—you would probably gain weight. But people don't eat here every night; it's an occasion place."

If, when they are customers, chefs find most portions put before them to be outsize, is there any good reason for them to load up what's served from their own kitchens? Yes, sometimes, reasons Marcus Samuelsson. At his Red Rooster Harlem, Samuelson serves a dish called Yard Bird, which is fried chicken with some gravy over greens. It's a big portion—my husband and I shared it one day (along with a salad, a side, and dessert) and still had leftovers. I mention this to Marcus the next time I see him. "That Yard Bird—that's a lotta chicken," I say.

"Yes, and it should be," he answers. "Because our reference point for that dish is *comfort* and *home*."

For Samuelsson and his colleagues, serving food isn't simply about feeding people for wellness. They aim to provide a transporting experience, one that might have new or familiar tastes, one that is evocative of a particular place or a time. They aren't merely apportioning food; they are narrating a story.

"As a chef, you have to be a good storyteller," he says. Thinking about a new dish, Samuelsson literally writes out a story, sometimes illustrated with pictures that he paints. He considers the neighborhood, both the people living there now and those who came before whose influences are still felt, however faintly. Where he lives and works, there is not only an African-American population, but Latin, Caribbean, and some Jewish and Italian. The story of the Yard Bird is one of comfort food and of abundance in this community, where big celebrations meant big plates of food—not a story of dieting celebutantes poolside in Malibu.

"Certain dishes should be large and rich and voluptuous. Others should be smaller, and balance that," he says. "Like, the taquitos are not big."

If you've never had the Yard Bird or the taquitos, how would you know? "You should ask!" says Samuelsson. "Everything is an opportunity to have a conversation. That's dining. Everything else is eating." So enjoy the stories that chefs tell through food. But don't feel shy about abridging them once in a while.

Lesson 52: **They separate value from appetite**

If you've been served double what you know you should eat, it takes some training to hold back. "Your first instinct is, 'I just paid eight dollars for this burrito, so I'm going to eat the whole thing,'" says Nate Appleman. "How many times have you finished a meal because you were 'paying good money'? Now I don't do that. But that's definitely a struggle, you know, because it's so ingrained in you."

Well-known chefs also have the opposite problem: They seem to attract free food whenever they sit down. They complain about it, but they do it to one another—sending over generous, showstopping dishes is a standard practice in chef society. "I used to finish everything. Now I try to eat until I'm full, then stop. It's just a matter of self-control," says Marc Murphy, who claims he tries not to perpetuate the practice, serving friends only what they order; but he does send desserts.

I listened to a lot of chefs hold forth on the subject of the free-food assault. Eric Ripert tends to cut overly generous friends off at the pass, by speaking to the waitstaff: "I am always very up-front. 'Please say to the chef not to be offended. I'm going to eat light.'" Here's Ming Tsai's take: "You're rude to not finish the short rib he sent out, so you have to say, 'Please wrap it up; I'm just stuffed.' I feel bad if they ask, 'Didn't you like it?' I say, 'No, I loved it. It's great. It's too much food.'"

Yeah, okay. That hardly ever happens to most of us. But even when you are paying for your dinner, you can still get slammed with too much food when the portions are out of whack. If you find it hard to hold back in those situations, well, maybe consider eating elsewhere. During his weight loss Art Smith says he really had to look at what triggered overeating, and choose restaurants "where people respect the fact that I'm on this path. I want to go out and dine, but I want to also feel that I'm not going to be assaulted by food. Food is love, but let people choose how they want to be loved."

There are other free-food hit-and-runs in nonchef lives. The box of doughnuts that sits seductively on the conference room table, calling to you after you've already had a better breakfast of yogurt and fruit, or the birthday cake offered when you came to pick up your child from another kid's party. I'm not suggesting you never partake of those unexpected treats, but it does seem worth spending a moment to ask yourself: Were you planning to stop and actually enter a doughnut shop or bakery and purchase a cruller or a slice of frosted layer cake today? If the answer is no, then why eat the free version that you didn't even ask for?

Lesson 53: They employ the takeaway

When Naomi Pomeroy opened Beast in Portland, she made a bold decision: six courses, no choices. With a prix-fixe menu that changes every week, "We really get to make what we feel like making," says Pomeroy. "People seem to trust us." As a result, this is not the place to go if you just want two appetizers or to substitute steamed vegetables. "It's nice to be in an atmosphere where people are celebratory and sort of let that stuff go," says Pomeroy. Then she laughs a little and admits, "At the same time, I've realized myself over the last couple of years that I can't let that stuff go myself."

Even at an "occasion" restaurant like Beast, it's okay, she says, to ask to have some food wrapped to take home. "I think it's smart. I like when I see people do that," she says. "Honestly, I couldn't eat all the food I serve at my restaurant."

She's also a big fan of leftovers herself. Besides being a check on portion size, "Leftovers means an extra twenty minutes of sleep in the morning, because I don't have to make lunch. I choose twenty minutes of sleep over extra calories any day."

Lesson 54: They don't eat "breakfast" when they sit down to dinner

A true story from Marc Murphy, which I will let him tell:

"Once when I went to L'Ambroisie in Paris, my friend was ordering in English, and the waiter said, 'Would you like the sauce on the plate?' So I said in French, 'Why would you ask us that? We're coming to a three-star Michelin restaurant; of course we want the sauce on the plate!' The waiter said, 'Oh, I wanted to check because a lot of Americans don't want the butter sauces.' Then he said, 'It's interesting, because they always ask for no butter sauce on the plate, but then before dinner they take the bread and they make the tartine!'" Here, Murphy demonstrates what the waiter was doing, miming the repeated slathering of butter on bread. "'I don't get it,' he said.

"It's true; in France a tartine is what you have with a cup of tea or coffee in the morning—a piece of bread, with a bunch of butter on it. That's breakfast. But before dinner you don't have three baskets of bread with butter or dipped in olive oil or whatever. Wouldn't you rather have the butter sauce? Leave the butter where it is supposed to be. The amount of butter in a butter sauce, what actually ends up on a plate, is not very much."

Thanks, Marc. Point taken. Allow the butter sauce on the plate where it belongs, and skip the buttered bread before dinner. If you can't resist the bread on the table, ask for a takeaway bag and have it, yes, for breakfast the next day.

Lesson 55: They have what she's having

Maybe a top restaurant in Paris isn't the place to start messing with the placement of the sauce. But is there ever a time and place when making a few alterations to a dish might be the best policy? Yes and no. Do chefs care whether you want it the way you want it, not the way they serve it? That depends, as we'll see.

Cat Cora travels a great deal, both for the Food Network and for her own restaurants and ventures. On the road, particularly outside of big cities, Cora says she applies a rule familiar to anyone who has seen *When Harry Met Sally*: "I'll order salad dressing on the side. I order sauce on the side—a lot of places put way more than you need. I don't go nutso over it, but I do customize for my health."

Recall that the waitress in the film rolls her eyes at having to adapt an order for the fussy Sally. But while some chefs institute a "no substitutions" rule on their menus, Cora—who has opened several eateries in extremely populist locales like Disney World and the San Francisco airport—is not one of them. "I don't mind. If someone doesn't want the starch, and they want steamed vegetables, fine. If they want sauce on the side, fine. Don't be afraid to custom-order your meal to how you're trying to eat."

Another way to think of it is uncoupling foods from their less healthy accompaniments. In a bistro, steak or mussels traditionally come with French fries. Just because that's the done thing doesn't mean you need to keep those pairings each time you order them. Even if a restaurant isn't thrilled to offer a substitute, just ask them to hold the fries—then order the vegetable side you want.

Myself, I'm a little timid about making substitutions, ever since more than one chef explained to me that, while they are willing to remove ingredients (when they aren't already integrated into a dish), they don't want customers telling them to add anything. "That's what we went to cooking school for," snapped one. So I was a bit surprised when I sat down at Art Smith's Art and Soul in Washington, D.C., ordered the Put-Ups Salad (studded with pickled vegetables), and was asked by the waiter whether I wanted to add a protein to that. Salmon? Shrimp? Chicken? None of this was on the menu, but it did make the salad more of a meal, and I was grateful for his having taken the lead.

Soon Art showed up and asked how I'd come to have salmon on my salad. Was I busted? Was the waiter? I told him what had gone down during the ordering.

"You know what?" he said. "The staff is buying into the fact that Chef Art wants people to have a choice and be healthy and be happy. That makes me feel good."

Despite some chefs' enthusiasm for the nixed potatoes or the added protein, be warned that this behavior won't go over well everywhere. At his first restaurant, the hip, clubby Father's Office in Santa Monica, Sang Yoon made a calculated choice of not honoring any requests for substitutions. With that policy, "We pissed some customers off," says Yoon. "But we pleased a lot more." (I ask you: Is there a better reassurance that you are a hip, adventurous diner than getting excited by a no-substitutions policy?)

Now, with his high-end Lukshon, he is slightly more flexible when it comes to omitting offending ingredients, "if we can leave it off without fundamentally altering the dish." But that doesn't happen often. Just last night, he tells me, "Someone asked if we could leave the Chinese sausage out of the black rice. That answer is 'no,' because the dish tastes completely different without it—it's naked. And a lady sat up there"—he indicates the stools that face into the open kitchen—"and said, 'Can't you just make me steamed spinach?' No. 'Well, I see you have spinach. Can't you just steam it?' It's not about 'can we.' It's just not what we do. It's not *who we are.*"

He would never say this to a customer, but: You can stay home and steam spinach. One of the pleasures of dining out is experiencing dishes you are unlikely ever to attempt at home. For Yoon, this is one of the pleasures of being a chef. "If someone with average skill could make the dish equally well, you probably shouldn't serve it in a restaurant. It's nice when you get a dish and you know 'that took a lot of labor, and there's a lot of love in that.' We have a dish that is baby Monterey squid, and we make a Chiang Mai–style sausage, stuffed inside, grilled and served with a 'pesto' with candlenuts and coriander too. If you look at it, you can see that's not something we just tossed in a wok, slapped together, and stirred it."

Yoon recalls years past, when he was working at Michael's in Santa Monica, where a power-player clientele felt the need to exercise control from the diner's seat. "It was literally 'make your own menu night' every night," he remembers. When the results of their customized orders didn't please them, he says, "They'd send it back. I'd be like, 'See?'"

From his perspective—and quite a few chefs share this view, even if they aren't as strident about it—the reason you're coming to his place is to experience the way he cooks food. Let him do his job, he reasons, and you're likely to enjoy it. You can go back on your diet tomorrow.

Lesson 56: They know tomorrow is another day

Sang Yoon's tough-love approach to service brings me to a final thought on the subject. Yes, you can and should substitute when you feel strongly that you need to and when you think you can get away with it. But otherwise, accept the fullness of what the chef has laid out for you—it is a gift to be enjoyed. Thomas Keller appreciates restaurants with a single, daily chef's menu—no choices—so that the decision-making is taken out of his hands. (His ad hoc restaurant works that way: Everyone gets the same meal, served family-style.) "If we have confidence in the chef, we should be happy with what they are going to make for us," says Keller. "In a way, you remove all anxiety by removing choice." Faced with a conventional menu, even at his Bouchon Bistro, he can be flummoxed. "Should I have the chicken, or the steak? Or the special monkfish? The oysters or the lettuce? Or wow, look at the special sweetbreads. All these choices creates a little bit of anxiety."

Just a little bit, of course. When we spoke, Keller had recently had a meal there that had clearly been a source of great enjoyment. His days are often fueled by whole grains, vegetables and hummus and his working nights see dinner at 4:15 p.m. "Eating early is key for me," both for keeping up energy and maintaining weight. Yet there he was at eight o'clock, tucking into a steak au poivre, potato gratin, creamed spinach, wine, and a pear tart with vanilla ice cream. "I enjoy eating that way, I just don't eat that way every night," says Keller. "Everything in moderation. I eat the way I like to eat, and I eat the way that I think is a healthy way to live."

Those two ideas need not be realized during a single repast—you can eat mainly for health at lunch, and purely for pleasure at dinner. "You can't count calories when you're out," says Karen Hatfield, pastry chef and co-owner of Hatfield's in L.A., with her husband, Quinn. "Our philosophy is: If you're going to eat it, eat it. If you're going to have a cappuccino, have whole milk in there. Not that you show no restraint, but you have to be able to eat." She and Quinn see food as energy when it's called for, but also as entertainment. Plus, she says, pulling a chef's trump card: "Going out to eat is part of our job."

Even if, as civilians, we can't justify a major meal as occupational research, there are a dozen other reasons to give in to the pleasure of a beautifully cooked and presented meal. The fruit and green tea will be waiting for you the next morning. You can eat salad for dinner an extra time that week. The gym will be open basically forever. So just go for it once in a while. Quinn Hatfield adds that between their busy work lives and new parenthood, it isn't as if they are swanning through a different Los Angeles restaurant every night. When the planets and the babysitter align, "We have to have a complete experience. We get the tasting menu. Or we get three courses. We're not going to hold back. We just have to demonstrate more restraint during the rest of our day."

Having lost eighty pounds, Michael Psilakis is very conscientious about how he eats during the week. When he started his weight-loss regimen he built in one night per week to go out and relax his rules. Initially on those days off, he ate anything he wanted. "Anything. I said, 'I'm going to have appetizers *and* entrées. I'm going to eat dessert; I'm going to eat ice cream. I'm going to go to the movies and eat candy if I want.'" But what he found was that the free-for-all wasn't undoing his continued weight loss so much as it was making him feel bad. "If you moderate what you eat all week long, at first you're so looking forward to that day off that you eat so much you feel horrible. The next time you won't want to feel horrible again, so eventually they just become little treats, not these big elaborate events."

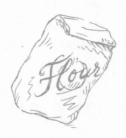

Melissa Perello's Spring Vegetable Salad with Creamy Herb-and-lemon Dressing

This is a perfect salad to eat for lunch the day of, or the day after, a night out. The generous use of aioli (garlicky mayonnaise) and crème fraîche or sour cream prevents it from becoming so austere as to make you feel as if you are doing penance.

serves 4

DRESSING

   ½ teaspoon anchovy paste
   ½ cup homemade aioli (or store-bought mayonnaise
      plus 1 clove garlic, very finely minced)
   ¼ cup crème fraîche or sour cream
   Juice and zest of 1 lemon*
   2 tablespoons chopped tarragon
   2 tablespoons chopped chervil
   1 tablespoon chopped parsley
   1 tablespoon minced fresh chives
   Salt
   Black pepper

*Melissa recommends two Meyer lemons here; they are smaller and less sour than the standard variety. If you can find them, use them.

1. In a small mixing bowl, combine the anchovy paste with the aioli (or mayonnaise and minced garlic).

2. Stir in crème fraîche or sour cream.

3. Add lemon juice and zest.

4. Stir in chopped herbs, then season to taste with salt and black pepper.

SALAD

> 4 small heads of gem lettuce or 2 to 3 romaine
>   hearts, leaves torn by hand
> 1 generous handful pea shoots (left whole if they are
>   small and tender, or leaves only if they are larger)
> 1 cup shelled and blanched English peas (or frozen
>   peas)
> 1 cup sliced and blanched asparagus or other green
>   vegetable, such as broccoli or green beans

1. In a large bowl, toss the lettuce, pea shoots, peas, and asparagus.

2. Gently fold in enough of the dressing to generously coat everything.

3. Season to taste and serve immediately.

Adapted from Melissa Perello.

Quinn Hatfield's Maine Lobster with Summer Succotash

"My parents were old-school foodies," says Hatfield, who was raised in North Carolina by Francophile parents. "They liked to go to restaurants and, if they ate something they liked, try to make it at home." That makes sense with a luxury item like lobster: It can be had much more inexpensively from the fishmonger (especially during a plentiful year) than it can with a restaurant's markup. Because it is usually served with a kiddie pool of butter, lobster has an undeserved reputation. In fact, it is lower in fat and calories than most meats and is high in omega-3s. But the real star here is the succotash, which doesn't take much time or effort, save for shelling the fava beans. (No one will turn you in if you use lima beans or edamame instead.) The succotash would also be good served with shrimp or scallops, or made ahead for a summer picnic.

serves 2

> 2 cups fava beans, shelled, or 2 cups lima beans or
>   edamame (thawed, if frozen)
> Kosher salt
> Two 1- to 2-pound Maine lobsters
> 3 large ears sweet corn
> 2 tablespoons butter (or olive oil)
> 1 cup cherry tomatoes, cut in half
> 12 basil leaves
> Black pepper

1. If you are using fava beans: Bring a medium pot of water to boil. Blanch the fava beans for two minutes, then drain. When they are just cool enough to handle, slip off the skins. This step can be done a day ahead, and the peeled beans stored in the refrigerator. (If using lima beans or edamame, skip this step.)

2. Fill a 4-gallon-capacity stockpot with 2 gallons of water, cover with a lid, and bring to a boil. When boiling, add enough kosher salt for the water to taste well seasoned (about ¼ cup—don't burn your tongue tasting). Add the lobsters and boil for 8 to 9 minutes for a one-pound lobster, 15 minutes for a two-pounder. When they are done (they will be bright red, and an antenna will pull off easily), remove the lobsters and allow to rest 5 to 10 minutes. Before serving, remove the meat from the shells.

3. Meanwhile, stand each ear of corn on end and remove the kernels by slicing down the side, then rotating and repeating. Doing this in a wide, shallow bowl or roasting pan with a towel in the bottom helps catch the kernels, protects your knife, and stabilizes the corn.

4. In a large sauté pan, heat the butter over medium-high heat until foamy and hot. Add the corn and season with salt. Cook, stirring occasionally, until the corn is tender and slightly caramelized, about 8 minutes. Add the peeled fava beans (or limas or edamame) and cook another 3 to 4 minutes until tender and bright green. Toss in the cherry tomatoes.

5. Tear the basil leaves into small pieces by hand and add to the pan. Season to taste with salt and a few grinds of black pepper, if desired, and serve the succotash immediately with the lobsters.

Adapted from Quinn Hatfield.

BEHIND THE LESSONS:

Michelle Bernstein, Knife in Hand

Saturday brunch was meant to be the calm before the storm.

It is the morning of the third day of the Wine & Food festival, and Michelle Bernstein will later tonight be hosting an event in which hundreds of diners will arrive simultaneously at her stately yet cool Miami Design District tapas restaurant, Sra. Martinez. (Her husband, David Martinez, is the co-owner.) Earlier, when I asked whether I might stop by, she told me to come on over, that brunch wouldn't be too crazy-busy. But something has changed.

Rick Bayless, headed home to Chicago after two days of events, has shown up with some of his staff for lunch on his way to the airport. Bernstein is apologetic as she explains to me that our chat will have to wait, and picks up her knife—she is going to handle this meal herself. Not a problem, I tell her. Can I watch? As long as I am out of the way in the restaurant's efficient if small kitchen. I wedge myself into a sliver of room next to the door frame and drop my bag on top of a freezer.

Bayless doesn't order from the menu; it is up to Bernstein to put together a lunch to impress without looking like she is trying to, that will satisfy without being too much before a flight. Oh, and Bayless is in a bit of a rush.

Standing in the crook of her L-shaped stainless counters, Bernstein, in a cobalt apron, is both conductor and first violin, chopping greens at the same time she is listening to the subtly changing sizzle in one of her cooks' pans, and letting him know it's time to get something off the heat. Then, as she continues to expedite brunch for all the other customers (she notices a dessert going out that she says looks "depressed" and orders a do-over; the second one is decidedly perkier), she puts together a menu for Bayless's table.

As first plates are ready, she inspects and finishes each one. An appetizer of small eggplant coins, fried and drizzled with honey and salt. Then razor clams with pata negra (Iberian ham) broth. A signature Bernstein dish: egg-yolk carpaccio, which is the improbable combination of yolks whipped with olive oil, briefly baked so it keeps a raw "carpaccio" brightness, and topped with shrimp and crispy shoestring potatoes.

Bernstein recalls how her mom, a Jewish-Argentine immigrant to Miami, used to pull elaborate and varied dinners seemingly out of the air. "It was amazing. To this day, I'm not sure how she did it. It was a different meal every night, but always at least five different dishes of salad, vegetables, a protein of some kind, a starch of some kind. Roast chicken to lasagna to gnocchi with braised chicken thighs to paellas. It was literally anything goes. It was food you'd find in a two- or three-star restaurant, even though she wasn't trained," Bernstein tells me during a separate interview. "I was always the last person at the table. When everyone else got up to do the dishes, I was still picking at the food. I always had a huge love for her food. She made salads in a huge plastic salad bowl, and I remember at the end of every dinner, I'd be the one to finish the salad, dipping my bread into the vinaigrette. I'm talking four or five years old."

That's the sort of satisfaction she's looking to deliver: the sopping-up-the-sauce-with-bread kind. Throughout the meal she is cooking for Bayless, Bernstein is serious and focused, though she occasionally checks in with the restaurant manager, who ducks into the kitchen with dispatches from the VIP table: They are eating everything, plates coming back empty. She allows herself a moment to exhale. "What else should we send them?" she asks aloud.

A rich stew of garbanzo beans, chorizo, spinach, and tetilla cheese goes out. Then white gigante beans with foie gras–duck sausage.

When the manager comes back with word that Bayless and company would like one more dish, then dessert, Bernstein sets to it, but not before arching an eyebrow and noting with a smile that this party was supposed to be in a hurry to get to the airport! She sends out a few more items before going out herself to say hello. Is there a meal that can ever prepare one to leave a clear, hot day in Miami for Chicago in February? This one came close. Later, from the car, Bayless tweets happily: "Just had the BEST meal @sra. Martinez."

Bernstein returns and notices me in the corner by the freezer, still taking notes and snapping photos manically on my phone. Of course, she wants to feed me. I give up my perch in the kitchen and take a seat in the dining room. The light, crispy eggplant rounds with honey are beautiful. I had watched them go past earlier, and thought of plucking one from the dish. Then her tangy, peppery take on shrimp cocktail with avocado and popcorn. A plate of pickles, briny and beautiful. I feel totally taken care of, and am somehow able to put the thought of all her hard work in the small room behind this one out of my mind, and just enjoy. Which is, I think, exactly why chefs do what they do.

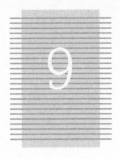

EAT DESSERT

STRICTLY SPEAKING, HUMANS don't require dessert in the same way they do protein or vitamins. Yet people talk about "needing" a little something sweet at the end of the day. Many of the same chefs who insist they delight mainly in savory foods nonetheless get near-rhapsodic about desserts they have known. To pick on one, let's take Ming Tsai, who once worked as a pastry chef in Paris under macaron king Pierre Hermé. "If I'm going to use up calories I'd rather have savory," he starts to tell me. Then: "But a really good cheesecake from New York? Absolutely. Oh, and I had the best doughnut recently, and pâte à choux filled with a marshmallow mascarpone cream; I ate, like, ten of those. So, yeah, every now and then."

Rick Moonen tells me something charmingly relatable: "Growing up I was chubby and I did some whacked-out shit: I'd eat chunks of brown sugar, or we would challenge each other to eat a tablespoon piled high with cocoa, and you'd turn it into fudge with the saliva in your mouth—you would laugh and powder would come out your nose." But in recent years, says Moonen, he's all but sworn off sweets. "I don't like what sugar does to me," he says. Mark Bittman doesn't eat sugar during the day, and Nate Appleman limits treats to Sunday with his son. But never having dessert doesn't work for anyone. Life is meant to be sweet.

Lesson 57: Smart chefs eat chocolate

By this I do not mean brownies, or chocolate-glazed doughnuts, or hot fudge on your ice cream. The number one sweet among chefs who spoke with me is straight-up dark chocolate, usually in bar form. Several said roughly the same thing: "Give me a really good piece of bittersweet chocolate." Or, "Just a square of dark chocolate," a square meaning the variably sized piece of a bar they can feel good about eating in one sitting. This is certainly a reasonable way to enjoy something sweet without causing major caloric destruction. Even Art Smith, who, as someone living with diabetes, is extremely conscientious about how much sugar he eats, says, "I still have chocolate every day." As for other desserts, he advises, "You have to say to them: 'Yeah, you're a friend of mine, but you can't visit often.'" But a small amount of dark chocolate (with a high percentage of chocolate and a lower percentage of sugar) gets a pass from nearly everyone.

Here's my one issue with the "just a square" proposition: I may need only a square, but when I'm holding the other seven squares in my hand . . . I want them too. Mark McEwan is with me on this: "You could not unwrap a large chocolate bar near me and not have me finish it," he says. "I'm not capable of not eating it."

As a compromise, you could buy those individually wrapped bite-size chocolates, but here's a better solution: more chocolate. Eric Ripert keeps a well-stocked supply of high-quality chocolate bars on the credenza in his office. "You will freak out when you see how much chocolate I have," he says. I take a peek: It's an impressive stack, with a dark chocolate–pink peppercorn bar balanced on top.

I soon understood that the idea of polishing off, in one sitting, the supply of chocolate bars in Ripert's office is absurd. So I started buying more chocolate, keeping three bars at a time in the cupboard. Shared with my husband and son, the chocolate actually lasted more than a week, enjoyed slowly and communally, a few squares at a time each night.

Which is not to say that the bars didn't sometimes call to me during the day when I was home writing, and I found myself having an inner dialogue that sounded very much like actual conversations I've had with my actual child. It usually took place around four p.m. and sounded (silently) something like this:

"There's chocolate in the cupboard. Can I eat it now?"

"No, the rule is chocolate at the end of the day. If you eat it now, you won't be able to enjoy it then. And you know you are going to want it."

"Right." Pause. "Can I eat it now?"

"No. But I promise you can have a piece later."

"Okay. Later."

Then I would forget about it. Before you get really worried about me, those conversations in my head ended as soon as I internalized the after-dinner chocolate rule. I actually stopped craving it at any other time. It helped to know that, as in Eric's office, there was always a supply. I had a little bit, and put the rest back and revisited it another night. You know what? It was never not delicious.

Lesson 58: They battle temptation by occasionally giving in

If you have to work on your birthday, is there a better assignment to have than to go to Jacques Torres's chocolate store and interview Mr. Chocolate himself?

I dare not tell Jacques it is my birthday. Last time I came to visit him with my son in tow, we left with a three-foot-tall milk-chocolate Easter bunny and a small retinue of ten-inch rabbits—all of which we had made, with Jacques's guidance, after donning hairnets and white lab coats. (The big bunny went to an Easter party at a friend's church, but the three of us carved off pieces of the smaller ones after dinner for many days running. Each night my husband would retell just the punch line of a fairly gruesome joke: "A pig that special, you don't eat all at once.") Later Jacques will sweetly chide me, "Why didn't you tell me it was your birthday?" Self-preservation, that's why.

A few years earlier, Torres was about thirty pounds heavier. You might think that working around pastry and chocolate for thirty years might have been the inevitable cause of his weight gain. But Jacques is fairly restrained around chocolate, preferring dark to milk, and pure chocolate over loaded confections. We settle into a table in the café area of his Hudson Street location. Is he as distracted as I am by the toasty perfume of cocoa in the air? Perhaps working around it all the time, he doesn't even notice anymore.

"Can you smell that?" I ask.

"Yes, we are making chocolate today," he says. "We have five hundred kilos of fresh chocolate. We just roasted the beans and it's ready, so today it is smelling a bit more." He is almost apologetic. I am swooning. This is really one of those places where you tell yourself: *If I worked here, I would gain weight.* How does he not?

"I certainly eat more chocolate than normal people," he tells me. He'll pick at dark chocolate, or nuts if they are coming out of the roaster. His biggest weakness is ice cream fresh from the churn. "Yes, this is a problem, because if I pass in front of the freezer when the ice cream comes out, I'm going to get some. It's the best time to eat ice cream. It's magic." Despite occasionally giving in to the call of fresh ice cream, Torres sounds a common refrain: "Having a passion to make chocolate doesn't mean eating chocolate all day." Because he can have wonderful sweets whenever he wants, he doesn't crave them in the same strong way a layman might when entering one of his stores.

Home is another story. In the evening, Torres is one of us. "You watch TV and you think, 'Do I have anything sweet?' So I keep no sweets in my apartment. And believe me, I could make some pretty good sweets." We are sitting next to a column stacked with some of his signature treats: small cellophane bags of dark chocolate–covered cornflakes and milk chocolate–covered Cheerios. For a guy who grew up with the French no-between-meals eating rule, he has certainly mastered the American art of making snack food. "I would not bring this in my home," he says. "If you open a package, you finish it. I don't go there." When he is forced to test his will, he admits defeat. Last weekend he brought home eight cookies, expecting eight guests, but there turned out to be only five. What became of the extra three cookies? Torres admits, as if even he is surprised by what happened next, "For breakfast, I had cookies!"

After our interview, Jacques asks whether I'd like a hot chocolate. This I cannot resist. It is, after all, my birthday.

Lesson 59: If having a little sugar leads to having a lot, smart chefs avoid it

Torres has figured this out for himself: Don't bring home the cookies/chocolate/ice cream, and you won't be tempted to finish off the whole package. But what to do when you live with someone who, infuriatingly, can eat one spoonful of ice cream and put the rest of the pint back in the freezer until tomorrow night?

From a gastronomic standpoint, Karen and Quinn Hatfield have a mixed marriage. "I'm the moderate in the family," says Karen, the pastry chef and manager of the Hollywood restaurant they own together, Hatfield's. "Quinn is the all-or-nothing guy. You can't give him ice cream, because he'll eat the whole container. But he can go without ice cream, whereas I love a little taste, and can have just a little bit."

It's true, her husband confirms. "I'm a huge sugar junkie. I'd be eating candy all the time. That's something I have to try really hard not to do." Though Quinn now has the physique of a competitive cyclist, back when he was building his career in New York he was heavier and felt he needed to do something about it. "The thing that clicked for me was watching my sugar," says Quinn. "I lost forty pounds."

Though she says nothing when she hears this, Karen's face indicates that she doubts his claim. Quinn counters, citing the numbers, "I went from 210 to 175."

"That's thirty-five pounds," she corrects with a smile.

Regardless, Quinn continues. "Eliminating sugar worked for

me. As I said, I have issues with sugar. If I wake up and eat my daughter's Gorilla Munch, then it's a sugar day and I eat sugar all day. If I go out to dinner, I'll eat every dessert on the table, go home, and feel bad about it. The next day, I won't eat any sugar."

"Really? None?" I ask.

Karen pipes up again, this time in his defense. "His self-control is very impressive. He can fast. He's done raw diets. For me, no. I have no desire to go to those extremes. I like sugar; I don't have a problem with it. When I'm working on a new dish, I have to eat it. So I might skip lunch that day." In part because she is disinclined to exercise with the same intensity as her husband does, Karen is careful to monitor and balance what she's eating, whether it's ice cream or other rich foods.

If she is going to eat dessert, Karen is really going to enjoy it. Here's what she likes: "Everything. Doesn't matter if it is fruit or chocolate or whatever. I like desserts made with skill, good ingredients, and balance." She's known for tempting diners with sophisticated roasted fruit cakes, and crowd-pleasers like chocolate–peanut butter truffle cake. "There are two schools of pastry chefs," Karen continues. "You'll encounter some who tell you they don't really like sweets. I am not down with that at all. I love it. It's no mystery why I got into this profession. I started messing around with this stuff at a very young age, and I haven't changed all that much. I like to bake; I like to see what other people have baked. I like it all."

Here's where it gets tricky for her husband and his sugar-avoidance plan. In their house, he says, "She's always got cookies, ice cream, some See's Candies. . . ."

"You're painting quite a picture!" She laughs. "Yes, I always have something. Not all of them at once."

"She's good about eating just two pieces of chocolate," he

says with a mix of admiration and envy. "For me, it was a matter of learning I just have to stay away from it."

Lesson 60: They know what they want (and why they want it)

As dessert is largely a "want" food, not a "need" food, if you're going to have it, have exactly what you desire. "I go straight for the chocolate," says Alex Guarnaschelli. "Go for the gusto, sit down opposite the food demon, look him in the eye, eat a block of chocolate, and move on. Don't kid yourself. Yes, I love fruit. But, *really*?"

Guarnaschelli tries also to be conscious of why she's reaching for something sweet. "Food is very personal, and very emotional. If I don't feel good or if I've had a crappy day, I'm going to have to 'quality-test' the chocolate sauce. That's no accident. It's hard not to say you deserve those things."

Sue Torres has a different approach to managing what she calls, only half in jest, her chocolate problem. "I've programmed my mind to go for the natural sweet. So I have at least a fruit a day, or fruit with yogurt to satisfy that need."

I have been trying to convince my son that fruit is an acceptable dessert. I'm sure I will be successful as soon as I convince myself of it. What I've been able to manage is a combination of Alex's and Sue's philosophies: Eat some fruit first, and if the chocolate is still beckoning, have a bit of that too.

If you are always ordering a berry tart because you think it is somehow more virtuous than the flourless chocolate cake that you really want (but never let yourself have), you may consume fewer calories, but will even those reduced calories be worth it?

"I won't bother with things I don't love," says Michelle Bernstein. Here's what's worth it, to her: "The Lady M's crepe cake in New York. It's probably one of the best things I've ever put in my mouth. I've had a birthday party in Miami and spent an exorbitant amount of money to order it. It's a cake of paper-thin crepes layered with pastry crème. You put that damn thing in front of me, and I'll eat it. I don't care. If I go to Joe's Stone Crab, I have to have a piece of key lime pie with a cup of coffee. But I go to Joe's Stone Crab maybe twice a year." This is a good test: If you can't describe from memory a dessert that you ate half a year ago, it probably wasn't worth having.

Though Bernstein rarely orders much dessert ("an espresso with sugar and a cookie after lunch is perfect"), somehow desserts find their way to her table when she dines out and is recognized by the kitchen. This, she says, is not—repeat, *not*—a crisis situation. "If they send me out a piece of cake, I'll eat the cake. I won't say no to the cake," says Bernstein. "Rather than think, 'I can't eat these things,' I think, 'Okay, I'll have a little cake now, and I won't have it later.' If I have it tomorrow, I won't have it for three days after. You have to compromise with yourself."

Lesson 61: They know how much dessert they actually need

When was the last time you went out to eat with friends and everyone ordered his or her own dessert? Never, right? Typically everyone gets his own dinner, his own drinks, and then as soon as the dessert menus are passed around, the sharing suddenly rivals that in group therapy. I'm in favor of sharing when it is to divide and conquer more of a menu. But dessert sharing is a pantomime of, "Oh, I couldn't eat another bite, but the brownie sundae looks pretty good."

Again, I'm going to defer to Chef Murphy, who has taken a bold stand on his menu: He offers only tiny desserts, too small to share. "If you go out with four people for dinner—what happens at the end? They share because nobody can eat a full dessert," he says. "But those two like chocolate; these two like crème brûlée. So what are they going to order, the chocolate mousse or the crème brûlée? Two people get stuck not having what they want. Or they order both and overeat and leave your restaurant feeling like shit."

His solution was to offer desserts that are very small. "You get your chocolate mousse, and I'll get my crème brûlée, and it's the right size—three bites. That's what a dessert should be, or you end up waddling out of there because you're so stuffed. You don't sleep well with all that sugar."

At Sang Yoon's Lukshon, the dessert is equally small, and free. "We give away dessert here," he says. "Why? First, most adults, with some exceptions, only want one or two bites of something sweet. Second, economically, most restaurants don't make any money on pastry. To sell dessert you have to remenu the table. 'Do you want anything? Should we share something?' The table is held hostage while you go through this big decision. So we have a pastry chef doing all great stuff, just miniature. It's like getting an *amuse bouche*, only at the end of the meal, when it has more impact and value."

The night I stop in with some friends, my dessert is a Vietnamese coffee custard with coffee streusel and condensed-milk ice cream, served in a shot glass. Just the right amount, though perhaps not for all of Lukshon's customers. "Some people say, 'Can I have more?' No," says Yoon. "We don't sell it. It's like a fortune cookie, or when you go out for Korean or Chinese food, you always get the four slices of orange. It's that symbolism, but ours is way better. They are gorgeous and rich, and it satiates that craving."

I think what he and Murphy are doing is perfect. But would everyone share my enthusiasm for the three-bite dessert? I took a classic chocolate mousse recipe—dark chocolate, butter, egg whites, sugar, heavy cream, and vanilla—that is intended to serve four and divvied it up into ten tiny ceramic sake cups. (I had some left over.) Those each hold about thirteen grams—much more reasonable than the 105 grams (including twenty-four grams of fat) in each original serving. Would my dinner guests agree, or would they think us crazy for serving miniature desserts? Too late now, I thought, while melting my chocolate bars in a bowl over simmering water and listening to the very fine first CD from France's first lady, Mme. Sarkozy. When our friends Mark and Kristina came over, I explained about tiny desserts. They liked the idea—especially Kristina. Everyone raved about the mousse. My son wanted another, so we let him have one. Once there were requests for more, it seemed miserly not to bring the rest out. So Mark had another. So did my husband. The last two little mousses sat in the center of the table while we sipped our decaf and kept talking. Eventually, Kristina and I began eyeing the remaining mousses. They were so small; what could having another one hurt? In the end, we ate more than we intended to. But it was only a first attempt, and I'm willing to try again. Tiny dessert in a restaurant is perfection; tiny dessert at home takes practice.

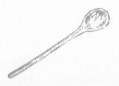

Jacques Torres's
Chocolate-covered Cereal

If you've never cooked with tempered chocolate before, you might believe you can skip that step and coat the cereal in merely melted chocolate. But in order to bring chocolate's fat molecules back into alignment for a shiny, snappy coating, you need first to raise the temperature of the chocolate (you can do this in the microwave), then lower it to just about 88°, and keep it there while working with it.

makes about 6 dozen clusters

> 4 cups very crisp cornflakes or other non-sugar-
>   coated cereal
> 1 pound bittersweet chocolate

1. Temper the chocolate: Place chopped, room-temperature chocolate in a microwave-safe bowl, preferably glass, and melt on high for 15 to 20 seconds at a time, until you have a slightly lumpy mix with about ⅓ of the chocolate still solid. With a rubber spatula, transfer the chocolate to a clean, cold bowl. Using a handheld blender (and a cooking thermometer, though not in the bowl simultaneously), beat the chocolate until it is smooth and the temperature has dropped to between 88° and 90°F (32°C). At this temperature, it is ready to work with.

2. Line two rimmed baking sheets with parchment paper.

3. Place the cereal in a large bowl and pour about half the tempered chocolate over the cereal. Using a rubber spatula, toss to coat evenly.

4. The chocolate will begin to cool and set. When the first coating has set, pour in the remaining chocolate and toss again to coat evenly.

5. Working quickly while the chocolate is still pliable, scoop small mounds of the cereal and place them on the baking sheets. Let stand for about 30 minutes, until hardened completely. If your kitchen is very warm, you can place the sheets in the refrigerator to speed the setting, but for no more than 10 minutes.

6. To store: Layer the clusters, separated by sheets of waxed paper, in an airtight container. Can be kept at room temperature for up to two weeks. (Author's note: If you are able to keep these around for two weeks, congratulate yourself on your willpower.)

Adapted from *A Year in Chocolate: 80 Recipes for Holidays and Special Occasions* by Jacques Torres. Stewart, Tabori & Chang, 2008.

—

Alex Guarnaschelli's Lemon-almond Cookies

Made with beaten egg whites, these cookies are delicate, delicious, and very easy to make.

makes 4 dozen cookies

> 2½ cups powdered sugar
> 2 cups almond flour
> 5 egg whites
> ½ teaspoon cream of tartar

1 vanilla bean, scraped (or 1 teaspoon vanilla extract)

Zest of 1 lemon

Nonstick spray

1. Coat 2 large baking sheets with a layer of parchment paper. Spray the paper with a thin layer of nonstick spray.

2. Preheat oven to 200°F.

3. In a medium bowl, sift together the powdered sugar and almond flour.

4. In the bowl of a stand mixer fitted with the whisk attachment, beat the 5 egg whites on medium speed for 1 minute to combine. Add the cream of tartar and beat the whites on high speed until soft peaks form, about 2 to 3 minutes. Add the scraped vanilla bean seeds and continue beating until it is fully incorporated and the whites are glossy, 2 to 3 minutes. Remove the bowl from the mixer and use a rubber spatula to gently fold in the lemon zest and the sugar–flour mixture.

5. Place heaping teaspoonsful of the batter about 2 inches apart on the prepared baking sheets. Take care to leave space between each cookie, because this batter spreads as it bakes.

6. Put the tray in the center of the oven and bake for 8 minutes; then raise the temperature to 375°F and bake until the cookies are golden brown around the edges and form a nice shell–like exterior, about 10 to 15 minutes. Remove from the oven and allow them to cool for a few minutes before carefully removing them from the tray.

Recipe courtesy of Alex Guarnaschelli.

Karen Hatfield's Apple Galette

"Having friends over is one of our favorite things to do," says Karen. Well, it was before they had two small kids. But even when it was just the two of them, they kept meals simple and rustic. "Quinn and I are kind of traditional—we're not home experimenting." She's also not a big home baker—her finely calibrated ovens and measuring instruments at the restaurant have spoiled her for the inaccuracies that can come with non-professional tools. She loves fruit tarts, though, and this one is easy enough for the amateurs among us to execute.

serves 4

FOR THE GALETTE DOUGH:

4 ounces (1 stick) cold butter
¼ teaspoon salt
1⅓ cups all-purpose flour
1 teaspoon sugar

FOR THE FILLING:

2 large (about 8 ounces each) Granny Smith apples
Granulated sugar for sprinkling
Melted butter for brushing

1. Cut butter into 2-tablespoon-size pieces and place in the freezer for 10 minutes. Measure the salt into ¼ cup cold water; stir well and place in the freezer for 10 minutes.

2. In the bowl of a food processor, place the flour and sugar. Pulse to combine. Remove the lid, add the butter, and pulse to combine until the butter is pea-size. With the motor running, stream in the water. As soon as all the water has been added, turn the motor off and scrape down the sides of the bowl. Pulse until the dough just comes together. Wrap in a large piece of plastic wrap and chill for at least 2 hours.

3. Preheat oven to 400°F. Roll out between 2 sheets of parchment paper until the dough is about ¼-inch thick and almost 10 inches in diameter. Keep refrigerated on a parchment-lined baking sheet until ready to use. Meanwhile, peel and core the apples. Slice the apples thin, about ⅛-inch thick. Sprinkle 1 to 2 tablespoons sugar over the bottom of the dough. Arrange the apple slices on top of the dough in a circular fashion, overlapping the slices just slightly. Using a pastry brush, brush the apple slices generously with melted butter and sprinkle with sugar. Bake until apples have browned slightly and the dough is fully cooked and lightly browned, about 35 to 40 minutes.

Adapted from Karen Hatfield.

Gregory Gourdet's Spice-roasted Stone Fruit

"Work takes up twelve hours of my day, so cooking at home has to be quick and easy—including dessert," says Gregory. "This dish is packed with ripe fruit and big flavors." It is also vegan. (He likes to serve it with a nondairy coconut ice cream.) This works well with any summer stone fruit; or in fall with pears. Don't leave off the last drizzle of olive oil or the chili flakes.

serves 4

4 to 5 ripe, fragrant plums or other fruit, washed,
   pitted, and cut into eighths

6 tablespoons agave nectar

½ ounce fresh gingerroot (about a 1-inch knob),
   peeled and cut into thin matchsticks

1 tiny pinch red chili flakes

Olive oil

Sea salt

4 cinnamon sticks

4 whole star anise

Zest of 1 lime

Nondairy coconut ice cream (optional)

1. Preheat oven to 425°F.

2. Coat the inside of a small (8-inch square or similar) ovenproof dish with a very thin layer of oil.

3. In a medium bowl, toss plum slices with agave, gingerroot, and chili flakes. Place in the prepared baking dish and drizzle with olive oil and a tiny pinch of salt. Place the cinnamon sticks and star anise over the plums.

4. Roast until soft and caramelized on the edges and juices thicken, about 30 to 40 minutes. Let cool to just warm.

5. Divide the plums, avoiding the sticks and stars, among 4 dessert bowls. Finish each with a sprinkle of sea salt, a rasp of lime zest, the ice cream (if using), and a drizzle of olive oil.

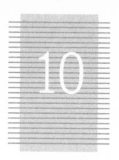

EAT AND DRINK
THOUGHTFULLY

IT WOULD BE a serious omission to talk to chefs about eating, and leave out drinking. Going out after the restaurant closes is an ingrained part of chef social life. "Alcohol is a big problem. Our business means at midnight we are talking, drinking, eating—and sometimes singing," says Masaharu Morimoto, a karaoke fan. I recall a memorable night at a New York charity event at the Harvard Club where Morimoto took the stage for a sing-off with Ming Tsai, who was clearly at a disadvantage, as the lyrics were in Japanese (and he was a Yalie at the Harvard Club). Still, a good time was had by all.

But that was rare, a party specifically organized for after midnight. Most nights the eating and drinking late is just a response to being let out from a job when the rest of the world is winding down. "I used to hate when I got off of work at one a.m. as a line cook: 'What do we do now?'" recalls Marc Murphy of his early years in the business. Most chefs who have ever struggled with unwanted pounds admit that they took on some of that extra weight in liquid form. "The biggest problem in the industry is that our downtime is midnight to four a.m.," says Murphy, "and nothing good goes on after midnight."

Lesson 62: Smart chefs don't drink like they used to

I begrudge no one his youth, but I wasn't particularly interested in hearing from chefs in their twenties who can go wild at night and wake up not only feeling fine, but knowing that all they have to do to avoid putting on weight is to keep up the usual set of unconscious metabolic processes. Get to a certain point, and something's got to give. Here's the math, courtesy of Tom Colicchio: "There are roughly two hundred calories in a cocktail. If you have five, that's a thousand—nearly half your calories for the whole day, which you've already eaten."

It may be an obvious point, but to weigh less, you may have to drink less. Morimoto proved that theory when he stepped on the scale a few years back and saw it nearing a hundred kilos (about 220 pounds). *I don't want to be a hundred kilos!* he thought, and immediately took action. He dialed back both the post-work drinking and the late-night bowls of ramen or Korean barbecue, and ramped up his workouts, lost forty pounds in three months, and, he says, felt much better.

Here's how you know that a lot of partying is a young chef's game, and when to get out of it: When Morimoto considered the reasons to lose weight and get healthier, he didn't think only of himself. "This restaurant has two hundred employees. It is called *Morimoto*. If I am doing something bad for my health, it is not going to be great business here. So I decided to move on," he told me. He still has a drink from time to time. "I still love karaoke and barbecue, but I am so busy that it's a struggle to find the time," says Morimoto. "That might be a good thing, though, as whenever I karaoke, I drink alcohol, because drinking is part of karaoke culture. So to stay healthy, it's good to keep yourself busy!" Happily for anyone who stumbles into the right karaoke bar at the right time, he hasn't given up singing either.

Some chefs have stopped consuming alcohol entirely, for reasons that go beyond the scale. "I got that out of my system when I was younger," says Nate Appleman, who appears to miss it not at all. When Alex Stratta began a reboot of his eating, he dropped all alcohol, and "that made a huge difference," he says. "It's a lifestyle consideration. I liked to indulge in everything, so I just abstain. If I have a glass of wine, I don't feel good. I love wine, but I've had my share."

Same with Gregory Gourdet. "As a personal choice, I don't drink at all," says Gourdet, though he's not advocating for everyone to do the same. "I have a lot of respect for wine. Wine has tons of antioxidants and health benefits, and it definitely enhances a dining experience. But I stopped, and that's helped me save on calories. I used to really enjoy small-brewery beers, but those pack a lot of calories as well, so it's something you need to factor into your meal if you're really watching calories and health. Fruity cocktails, which can be fun in the summer months, are way too high in sugar. As fun as they taste, it's good to be cautious with those. But, obviously, nothing in moderation is going to kill you."

Plenty of chefs who still enjoy a drink know this, and have curbed their behavior. Leave the multiple mixed drinks and fruity cocktails to the young. Easier said than done for some. There are few things that feel more hospitable than a specialty cocktail offered when you enter a party; I have trouble saying no to one. But I have no trouble saying no to two.

Lesson 63: They drink water

In grade school back in Dayton, Ohio, Ming Tsai played tennis and dreamed of going to Wimbledon. Despite being so active, he claims that as a preteen he was "a little chubby." So the ten-year-old Ming came up with his own regimen to get lean. "It basically consisted of doing one hundred sit-ups every day, and drinking six glasses of water before every meal."

The sit-ups-and-water routine lasted about a year, and had less of an effect than did shooting up six inches as an adolescent. But Ming has retained one element from his younger self's well-intentioned plan: drinking water before drinking anything else. "If I go to New York or I'm out partying with all my chef friends, I will drink a full glass of water with every alcoholic beverage I drink," says Tsai. "One for one, that's my secret." If you can't drink any more water, you're probably done with the hard stuff too.

In addition to slowing down one's alcohol consumption, water is the perfect beverage to replace soft drinks, which typically fail the real-food test—they are full of corn syrup or artificial sweeteners. Giving those up was crucial to Art Smith's new way of eating and living. "I can't *tell* you the evils of diet soda," he says over lunch. "Honey, I quit drinking diet soda, and now I drink a lot of water. In eight months I have not had a diet soda in my mouth. I have not had Splenda in my mouth. I have not had NutraSweet in my mouth. I don't even have stevia [an herbal sugar substitute] in my mouth. I have none of that, be-cause it creates bingeing; it makes you hungry. If there was one key to my weight loss, it was learning to look at something as beautiful as a glass of water as not only a source of refreshment, but a source of health."

Lesson 64: **They try not to let alcohol pick the menu**

Going out after work usually means eating as well as drinking. "It's a lifestyle thing," says Naomi Pomeroy. "You don't have time to eat when you work late hours, so you're starving at midnight, which is a bad time to start eating. If you have one or two cocktails, not only is that extra calories, but it is bad decision-making time."

When she launched her restaurant, dinner was sometimes just bread with butter or olive oil. "That plus a few glasses of wine? Doesn't look good in a bathing suit," she says with a laugh. Up about thirty pounds from the weight at which she is comfortable, Pomeroy decided to make some changes. "Hon-estly, my thirty pounds was from drinking, not from what I eat at work."

Sometimes the drinking starts earlier. Says New York chef Simpson Wong, "On a busy night, friends come in; they want you to sit with them; they want to buy you a glass of wine. Other friends stop in, another glass of wine." His nights out are fewer, but he remembers going to Koreatown or Chinatown or someplace open late, like Balthazar, a round-the-clock bistro in SoHo. "After a few glasses, your judgment is all mixed up. I used to pick up a burger and fries, then go to sleep."

This is the corollary to eating with your eyes open: Don't let your vision get blurred. But it happens. After the very occasional night of excess, Wong, who typically doesn't each much breakfast, will make himself a hydrating soup. "Your body craves fluids," he says. "If I've gone out, the next day I take a jar of tom yum paste, a pot of water, fish sauce, glass noodles, and green vegetables. The soup makes me sweat, because it's spicy and sour and hot. I sit in front of the TV, watch CNN International, and sweat it out."

Lesson 65: They don't let the drinking start long before the dining does

There is a movie line that my husband likes to quote when things don't go exactly as planned. It comes from a touching domestic moment (involving a projectile frosted cake aimed at someone's head) in the 1986 action flick *Raw Deal*. So put on your best *Ah*-nold Schwarzenegger voice and say it with me: "You should not drink . . . *und* bake."

Am I the only person who pops open the wine bottle while I'm cooking? Surely not. Sometimes the recipe you are preparing at that very moment calls for wine or beer, and as long as it's open, right? But this all but ensures that you will sit down to a meal and pour yourself yet another glass (or two), having already downed one (or two).

Of course, if you're cooking alongside a friend, it just feels impolite not to offer, and then to let them drink alone. Ted and Matt Lee almost always cook together when they are testing recipes, inviting family and neighbors to enjoy and critique the results. For a while, they were also writing a wine column for a magazine. "People would send us wine," recalls Ted. "There was always some around, and you do have a mandate to taste wine, so why not have a taste at four p.m.? By the end of the evening, that's a bottle, and alcohol is a lot of calories and sugar."

So starting to drink before you've even gotten the food to the table isn't the way to go if you want to keep track of your intake. It's just extra calories that won't add to your enjoyment when you finally do sit down. Though Matt Lee has always been naturally slender, now that he is past forty he notices when what he consumes has an effect on him. "It's not the fats or the volume of food, but the carbohydrates in liquid sources that are the main threat," he says. "I've gotten rid of the four p.m. beer."

Lesson 66: Some smart chefs still enjoy wine with food

Consumed immoderately, wine "is a huge calorie builder," says Mark McEwan. "Four glasses of wine before you go to bed will give you a belly real quick." Yet as conscious as he is about how he eats and drinks, he still feels that, particularly over a meal with friends, "it's very engaging to kill a bottle of wine." Nearly across the board among chefs, wine is described as part of the pleasure of a good meal.

Throughout his weight loss, wine remained part of Joe Bastianich's job—he owns wineries in Italy—and his life. That is something he has no intention of reforming. He still drinks wine nearly every day, a glass or two either at lunch or dinner. I assumed that this was an occupational hazard. But he quickly disabuses me of that notion.

"My job is to taste wine and know wine and be a buyer of wine. My job is not to *drink* wine," he says. "I drink wine because I like it." How much he consumes is "moderated by what

I have to get up and do the next morning." That's a big switch from the early days of his partnership with Mario Batali. "We'd get a *côte* for two at Balthazar with three bottles of wine. It was celebratory eating after working hard. Do that for a couple of months and the weight jumps on you."

He's cut back, for sure, but sees no reason to give up wine entirely. "A glass of wine has 140 calories—even if you drink two, all you have to do is not eat a Snickers bar and you're at the same place." (Here's the math: A regular Snickers bar is two hundred and eighty calories, same as two six-ounce glasses of wine.) But, unlike candy bars, wine has an expansive effect on eating and drinking—it tends to make people do more of both. "And that's kind of life," he says. "That's the beauty of life: eating a good meal, having a couple of bottles of wine with friends, and laughing and being happy."

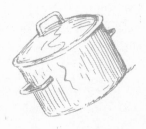

Simpson Wong's Hangover Soup

Wong describes this as a "kitchen sink" recipe—just throw in whatever you have. From experience, I know it can take leftover roasted chicken, kale, garlic, chives, scallions, and rice. The broth is delicious, and well worth preparing for breakfast—with or without a hangover—or any other time of day, if you're not into greens and fish sauce first thing when you wake up. But try them, try them and you will see. . . .

Makes one generous serving; you can throw in fewer ingredients, but keep the two cups of broth for a big, steamy bowl.

> 2 cups water or chicken broth
> 1 teaspoon store-bought tom yum paste (a widely stocked Thai spice paste, usually containing chili, garlic, lemongrass, shrimp paste, and galangal, a relative of ginger)
> ½ teaspoon sugar
> ½ teaspoon fish sauce
> ½ teaspoon lime juice
> ½ cup chicken breast (sliced thin)
> 5 shrimp (peeled and deveined)
> ½ cup vegetables
> 1 cup rice noodles (presoaked in cold water for ½ hour), or ½ cup of cooked rice
> 2 tablespoons chopped cilantro or scallions
> Salt and pepper to taste

1. Bring water to a boil; add tom yum paste, sugar, fish sauce, and lime juice.

2. Add chicken and cook for 1 minute, making sure chicken is cooked through.

3. Add shrimp, vegetables, and noodles. Cook for another minute. Season with salt and pepper to taste. Pour the noodle soup into a bowl; top with cilantro and serve.

Adapted from Simpson Wong.

━━

Mark McEwan's Steak with Horseradish Dressing

Horseradish and beef are a classic pairing, but McEwan's take isn't the traditional dairy-based creamy sauce. His sharp vinaigrette is terrific on the steak we tried it with, but would go great with fish or chicken, on sandwiches or potatoes. The recipe makes more than you'll need for four six- to eight-ounce steaks, so you'll have some left over for experimenting. Mark recommends pairing with a Chardonnay or Pinot Noir.

serves 4

⅓ cup white wine vinegar

3 tablespoons freshly grated horseradish

1 teaspoon Dijon mustard

6 parsley sprigs, roughly chopped

1 sprig fresh thyme, chopped

⅔ cup olive oil

Salt and pepper

4 6- to 8-ounce boneless, center-cut New York strip
    steaks, grass-fed preferred

1. Whisk together the vinegar, horseradish, Dijon, parsley, and thyme.

2. Whisking continuously, slowly add the olive oil in a thin stream. Season to taste with salt and pepper.

3. Preheat a grill over high heat.

4. Generously season the steaks with olive oil, salt, and pepper.

5. Cook over high heat for 3 to 4 minutes on each side for medium-rare doneness, longer depending on personal preference.

6. Let the steaks rest on a warmed serving platter, loosely covered with foil, for 10 minutes before serving with the horseradish sauce.

Adapted from Mark McEwan.

✦

Matt and Ted Lee's Shrimp Burgers

The Lees have surveyed shrimp burgers throughout the South's many shrimping towns, and developed their own take with lemon and ginger. A slightly oaky white wine pairs well. They also like a hoppy American ale with them.

serves 4

> 2 quarts water
> 1 tablespoon shrimp or crab boil, like Old Bay
> 1 pound headless large shrimp (26 to 30 per
>   pound), shells on

2 tablespoons chopped scallions

¼ cup fresh corn kernels, cut from the cob, about
    half an ear (or frozen, if it's winter)

2 tablespoons chopped flat-leaf parsley

1 tablespoon grated fresh ginger

1½ teaspoons lemon zest (from 1 lemon)

3 tablespoons high-quality store-bought mayon-
    naise, such as Duke's or Hellmann's

1 cup bread crumbs, preferably fresh (from about 2
    slices bread)

Kosher salt to taste

Freshly ground black pepper to taste

1 egg, beaten

1½ tablespoons canola oil

4 hamburger buns (optional)

Lettuce leaves

Tomato slices

1. In a 3-quart saucepan, bring the water and shrimp boil to a boil over high heat. Turn off the heat, add the shrimp, and let stand until they are just pink, about 2 minutes.

2. Drain and run under cold water to stop the cooking. Peel and devein the shrimp. You should have 1¾ cups chopped shrimp.

3. In a large bowl, mix the shrimp with the scallions, corn, parsley, ginger, and lemon zest. Stir in the mayonnaise and bread crumbs and season with salt and black pepper. Add the egg and gently fold with a wooden spoon or rubber spatula until evenly distributed.

4. Form the shrimp mixture into 4 patties, each 3 inches in diameter. Wrap the patties in plastic wrap and let stand in the refrigerator for 30 minutes.

5. Remove the burgers from the refrigerator and unwrap. Place the oil in a 12-inch skillet and heat over high heat. When it shimmers, add the burgers and sauté until gently browned, about 3 minutes per side. Drain on a dinner plate lined with paper towels.

6. Serve on toasted hamburger buns with lettuce, tomatoes.

Adapted from *The Lee Bros. Southern Cookbook: Stories and Recipes for Southerners and Would-be Southerners* by Matt Lee and Ted Lee. W. W. Norton and Co., 2006.

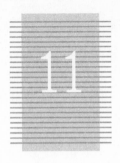

EAT TO FUEL
YOUR BODY

"YEAH, I EXERCISE," Nancy Silverton tells me, with an implied shrug over the phone. "But I'm no *Joe Bastianich*."

Bastianich has got to love that in the last few years he has become a benchmark by which others (or at least Silverton, one of his partners in two Los Angeles restaurants) can measure their physical activity. Bastianich's makeover from a soft-in-the-middle wine-and-food guy to a lean marathon runner is nothing short of modern legend in the food world; everybody asked whether I'd be talking to him about it.

I long debated whether to ask food folk about exercise. Phys ed is not their area of expertise, so consulting them about it didn't have the same logic as tapping their food knowledge. At the same time, if we are to talk about how chefs control their weight, it feels disingenuous to imply that they do it through dietary measures alone.

Once I began inquiring about their fitness regimes, I noticed a few things: First, many chefs approach their workouts with the same intensity and need for mastery that they bring to their work in the kitchen; some have even competed in their sports. This group has tailored how they eat to suit the demands of their activity.

A second group takes the opposite approach: They are tolerant of exercise and work out mainly to offset what they want and need to eat. By their own estimations, chefs will sometimes eat more than four thousand calories a day in the line of duty. Fortunately, because most normal people don't eat that much in a day, we need not aspire to be superathletes to compensate.

I've included stories of chefs who train intensively both because these testimonials inspire me ("if Art Smith can run twenty-six miles, surely I can run five. . . ."), and because they illustrate the physical exertion required to eat without boundaries. Far more accessible, and equally inspiring, is the example of chefs who work out by doing something they love to do, whether it's boxing, yoga, dancing, or running.

Some claim to avoid exercise. Matt Lee is one such infuriating soul. "I don't exercise at all," he reports, not so much a brag as a fact. "My activity is seasonal, gardening and home improvement stuff in the spring and summer."

Ted Lee, however, is an enthusiastic convert to working out. After a particularly well-fed summer in France, where his wife was an artist in residence at the Monet foundation, Ted decided to join a gym with her. "I love it. I realized I need to get my heart rate up. I feel like just as you balance your food, you need to balance your activities."

Lesson 67: Smart chefs run (and eat to run)

As a teen, says Joe Bastianich, "I was not what you would call 'athletic.'" In order to drop the sixty extra pounds he was carrying by his late thirties, he knew exercise had to be part of the equation. He started walking—the first day "was hell," he says. But he stuck with it and worked up to running, first a mile, then a 5K, then a 10K. The first time he finished the New York City Marathon was "a life-changing day." Running, even shorter distances, he feels "is magic. If you're lucky enough to be able to run, it will cure you of everything that's wrong in your life. It is that powerful."

While he is a model of what running can do (cure *everything* that's wrong? maybe not), Bastianich allows that getting to this level of fitness wasn't easy. "You have to deal with six months of pain," he says. In his experience, the endorphins—that famed runner's high—don't kick in until the fourth or fifth mile of a run, and many frustrated would-be runners give up before they can comfortably cover that distance. "They experience only the pain, and never get the pleasure of running." No one doubts Bastianich the wine expert when he talks about the pleasures of a glass of Friulano. He wishes they would trust him on the running thing too. "It really becomes a joy," he says. "Running the New York City Marathon is like being a seven-year-old on Christmas day."

At his level of training, he can basically eat anything—pasta, cheese, wine—without putting weight back on, and still enjoys a great meal with friends. But now he also thinks about which foods will power his workouts, and which will slog him down. "You have to eat commensurate with how you're asking your body to perform—you're looking at food as fuel. Before, food was a reward for a job well-done, or a way to entertain myself. Now I find other ways."

Just before his son Oliver's birth in 2007, Nate Appleman's weight reached "the pinnacle," 250 on the scale. (He's five-foot-seven.) "I gained baby weight as well. I was really big." He saw himself in a dire situation, but believed he could run the weight off; he didn't alter his diet at all—those changes came later. "I didn't know the first thing about working out or taking care of yourself. So I just ran. When I say 'ran' I mean I would run a block, then walk a block, then maybe the next week I'd run two blocks. The first time I ran a mile without stopping it was a huge accomplishment," says Appleman. Though he has since run marathons in less than four hours, he hasn't forgotten the feeling of those triumphant first blocks—and the pain and exhaustion that followed. "I had really bad shin splints, to the point where I wore braces and shin splint guards. I would come home and—this is before I got rid of my TV—I would fall asleep watching TV. When I would get up to go to bed, I could barely walk. That lasted a year." (News flash: Just as restaurant chefs don't eat the way they cook in restaurants, TV chefs don't necessarily watch a lot of TV. In my estimation, no one has ever become *less active* by getting rid of the box.)

Another chef who rethought his eating habits as he upped the intensity of his athletic challenges is Gregory Gourdet. A move to the West Coast from New York provided an opportunity for a clean slate. Although he hadn't exercised with any regularity since high school, "I started running. I was trying to figure what burned the most calories the fastest, and running was the easiest thing to do. I would get up and go a couple miles here and there. Then I got involved with people who ran more than I did, and I set goals for distances until I did my first half marathon. Then six months of training for my first marathon. Then ultramarathon: thirty-one miles, which was a six-hour run."

Soon he adapted his diet to support his training. He gets protein from eggs, fish, or chicken, eats loads of vegetables and fruits, and cut out dairy, red meat, most grains and beans, and alcohol. "I found I'm a lot faster when I'm on the lighter side," says Gourdet. "I was 185 to 220 pounds for most of my chef career, and now, training for my first triathlon, I stay 160 to 165. It makes a huge difference. But when the winter hits and it's cold outside, I'll gain ten pounds."

At his heaviest Art Smith hadn't wanted to walk around the block. By training with determination, he finished the Chicago marathon. When he married his boyfriend of ten years in 2010, the wedding began with the guests and the grooms running four miles through Washington, D.C. (Don't worry: They showered and changed before the party.) Yes, it was a little bit of a stunt, and it got some press, but it meant more people learned about Smith and his example of getting healthy. "I think when it comes to weight loss, regardless of whether you're a chef or not, you're just looking for some kind of inspiration. Losing weight takes more than willpower. It takes a great sense of support around you."

For Marcus Samuelsson, the motivation to run in Central Park comes from a different place. "I never thought about it from a 'working out' point of view; I think of it from a sanity point of view," he says. "I never think, 'I need to run six miles today because I've gained weight.'" Instead, he says, he is driven to carve out the time to clear his head, to think without distractions. "I need to be by myself. By mile two or three, I'm thinking: 'I wonder if the suckling pig should be done with jerk? Jerk is relevant for what we do at the Rooster, and I don't want to do suckling pig like everybody else does suckling pig. Should we serve that with pickled peaches—peaches have come in season. Yeah, let's do that. And mustard seed. Oh, no, we have mustard seed in something else. Take it out.' By mile five, 'Maybe we should do a fish?' And I think about my staff. 'Can this person take the step from line cook to sous chef?' I think about the sacrifices she's made, and what we've done to teach her. Running gives me a space to think about all that."

Simpson Wong, who jogs along the Hudson River, also subscribes to the idea of a moving meditation. "Running clears your mind," he says. "You have to empty the garbage can; then new ideas can come in. I love that."

Lesson 68: They work out to work off what they eat

"I came to a realization a long time ago that I'm never going to change the way I eat," says Michael Symon. "I cannot walk by the bread station and not eat a piece of bread. It's essentially impossible for me. So I work out five to seven days a week. It's the only way to counteract the calories." Symon, among those in the exercise-to-consume camp, was a wrestler in high school until he broke his arm. These days he meets up with a longtime friend in the gym. "We'll lift four days a week and do cardio two or three days. If I want to be in shape, that's how I have to live."

It's cyclical, of course: The more you eat, the more you need to work out, and the more you work out, the more you may feel you need to eat. This can totally undo your efforts if you reward yourself too often. But it can also change your relationship with food for the better. I don't aspire to be a long-distance runner, though my mother ran the Los Angeles Marathon when she was fifty-two, so never say never. The most I can handle so far is a 10K. Running, even at that length, stokes the appetite in a way that makes me hungry but not inclined to overeat. Dining after a good run has an element of reward for a job well-done, but also a built-in constraint: I don't want to sabotage my attempts at getting in shape. After an early fall race in Central Park I was hungry, sure, but I felt great and wanted to eat something as healthy as it was delicious. Breakfast was two poached eggs over fava beans at Morandi, the café in my neighborhood where I go for great Italian brunches and sightings of a breed of actors more often seen at the Sundance Film Festival. Were any there that day? Who knows. I was deep into my eggs.

Lesson 69: They play like they're still kids

A chef's hero is not necessarily another chef. As a boy in 1970s Hong Kong, Susur Lee idolized Bruce Lee, and asked his mom for kung fu lessons. "I used to go up the hill to school in the morning and see people doing martial arts, ladies and men, in the Communist outfit of blue pants, white shirts, and the braid with the ribbon. Even the women looked very masculine, but they would kick ass!" He soon got lessons and says, "I loved practicing. I was a very physical kid." His teacher also gave instruction in philosophy and calligraphy, which the students practiced on toilet paper "scrolls." "He told me, 'If you want to see farther, you have to climb more steps,'" recalls Lee. "I still have that scroll in my first restaurant."

Susur started dressing like Bruce Lee, wearing tracksuits everywhere; he was fifteen when the star died. "He was one of a kind, a master and a philosopher. Hardworking, so inspirational." That Bruce Lee excelled at many forms of martial arts, from kung fu to ju kwan do to aikido, impressed the teenage Susur. "I saw how if you mix things together, you make it yours, one of a kind. I thought of this when I started cooking; I wanted to know everything: chef, baker, wok chef—and be good at everything. Cooking reminded me of martial arts; it gave me the joy of being physical." So while he's no longer attending kung fu classes, those early days laid a foundation for a fit life. He plays tennis, runs, and more recently took up yoga and saw that "the warm-up is very similar to martial arts."

I think Susur offers a good example of getting in touch with the active children many of us—including the more sedentary among us—once were. Going to the gym can feel like a chore. But finding a sport or activity that harkens back to childhood can make physical activity a pleasure.

In addition to running, Marcus Samuelsson has played soccer since he was a boy. In his early forties, he says his game is still pretty good—he holds his own against twenty-one-year-olds. For him, soccer isn't just running around on a field; it is a weekly piece of home. He plays in a regular game in lower Manhattan with a group of Swedish ex-pats, none of whom are ethnic Swedes. "There's Iranian Swedes, Turkish Swedes, Jewish Swedes, Latin-American Swedes," explains Samuelsson. "We call ourselves 'Blatte United,' which refers to what we were called when we were kids—it was very negative. We've sort of converted it to celebrate that word, but we are also patriotic; we are all Swedish and living in America. We play against Brits, Germans, Brazilians, French. It's the biggest game in the world, but it is sort of underground in New York City."

This high-energy game is not the time to zone out and meditate on personnel issues or menu changes. "You can't when you've got someone running at you." But that change of venue is as essential as his time alone on the running track. "It's great, and it's a social experience with no cooking involved, which is important."

Sang Yoon has played hockey with intensity since childhood, through his years at Boston University. He still gets on the ice regularly in an adult league. The morning that we meet, he has just come from the dentist. "I took a puck to the mouth," he tells me. "See the scar? I knocked a tooth out." In the past, he says, "I've torn my ACL, torn my rotator cuff, torn a groin muscle, an abdominal muscle, and a ligament in my ankle, all in the last three years." During his rehab from one injury, he took up Pilates. Then he was back on the ice. "Hockey is something I want to do on an ongoing basis. I refuse to take up golf, or a safer activity. My parents ask, 'Why do you still do this?' Why? Because it's exciting! I like to skate more than I like to walk."

Lesson 70: They tap into a passion

As a teen Tom Colicchio was a jock of all trades: "Football, basketball, baseball, and I was a competitive swimmer from ages ten to seventeen." He also had always loved boxing—watching it, that is. "My parents were both fight fans," says the New Jersey native. A few years ago he was enjoying a bout at Madison Square Garden when he got a tap on the shoulder from a man who recognized him. "He said he was a trainer, and told me to give him a call if I ever wanted to work out. I did, and now I'm totally addicted to it."

No kidding. The first time I met Tom was at a magazine photo shoot with the *Top Chef* gang posing around a Thanksgiving table. While food stylists fake-cooked a turkey, and hair and clothing stylists whirred around his costars, Padma Lakshmi and Gail Simmons, Tom stood waiting, bemoaning his unnecessarily early call time. "I could be boxing right now." He sighed. "It's not like I need my hair done." At his peak he was in the ring three times a week—shadowboxing, working the bag, sparring, and going up to six rounds against his trainer. Wait, someone is getting paid to hit Tom Colicchio? In the face? (Does Bravo exec Andy Cohen know about this?)

"Oh, sure," Colicchio says. "You have headgear on, and my trainer is not trying to knock me out, just score points. But you get hit; it's the game." Absorbing punches aside, what appeals to him and other devotees about an activity like boxing (over, say, the treadmill) is that it engages not only the body but the mind. "It's like a chess match."

Music brings passion and purpose to Art Smith's workouts. On a trip to New York, when he had first started losing weight, a friend suggested he stop in at a particular Chelsea gym known for its body-obsessed gay clientele. Smith thought the idea preposterous—he was far too self-conscious to walk through the door there. Yet somehow he ended up in that gym, bringing his then pretty large self onto the floor alongside what seemed to him to be a roomful of hard bodies. He focused on the disco sound track drowning out any perceived slights against him. "Honey, I love to dance," he tells me. "When I heard that music I got on that elliptical and *I. Went. Crazy.* I loved it." Back at home in Chicago, he joined a branch of the same gym.

Music can make you do funny things. It can make otherwise sensible people in black-tie wedding finery do the Macarena. Smith found it was the same with exercise. Filling an iPod with the music he loved—and that means a lotta Lady Gaga—got him to move. "I think I lost eighty-five pounds from 'Bad Romance,'" he tells me. "I have my iPod on, and I play it loud, and I'm going to town. You find that happy place, and you go for it."

Simpson Wong got a musical infusion when he was visiting India. "It was holy season, and at the resort they gave everyone a white outfit and they had a celebration with different-colored powder that you throw at each other, and you dance to live Bollywood songs." Exhilarated by the experience, he sought out a studio that teaches Bollywood classes here in New York. "Dancing is great exercise. You move every part of your body. I like it a lot." That's really the key, isn't it? Find what you like a lot.

Lesson 71: **They get on their bikes**

For a certain type of person, it isn't enough to feed a passion at the amateur level; they want to compete with the pros. Under those conditions, a workout isn't about burning off last night's lasagna; it's about a person becoming the best he can be at his sport. Two chefs surprised me with their more-than-a-hobby approach to fitness.

While reaching the critical top of the Chicago food scene, Laurent Gras was simultaneously riding up to four hundred miles a week on his racing bike. Then Gras moved to New York with plans both to open a restaurant and to enter ranked competition. "I'll get a license from the U.S. cycling federation, join a club in New York, train with the team, and compete in the spring. That's the goal," he told me, adding, "besides looking for work." (That proved no problem; he became a popular guest chef and object of obsession for foodies who track temporary "pop-up" dining experiences.)

While this amount of exercise—he rides for five hours at a stretch—will incinerate anything Gras cares to eat, he is actually pretty mindful about eating exactly what his body requires. If he eats too much, he might carry extra weight; not enough and he will literally run out of fuel on a long ride. "You can blow out on the bike because you have no more power. I eat gels or bars on the bike." I find this just short of shocking, to think of this French chef eating unit doses of food-energy product. But this illustrates the difference between eating for pleasure and eating for exercise. When he's training, he says, he needs six to seven thousand calories a day (burning seven or eight hundred calories an hour). "You really do need a lot of food. I will eat a pound of pasta."

In the off-season he trains and eats like, I hesitate to say, a more or less regular person. "When I go to the gym and just exercise, I don't need to eat so much." As a result of his careful calibration, during training Gras keeps his body fat at about two percent—a distinction that earned him a place in the *Men's Fitness* 2010 lineup of the world's twenty-five fittest guys. (Irony alert: Gras is French for *fat*.)

On the other side of the country, Quinn Hatfield is equally bicycle-obsessed, but in a slightly different way. He competes in velodrome races that are over in seventy seconds or less. "I'm not a moderate guy," he reminds me. "I try to train as hard as I work." He's in Hatfield's kitchen from five to eleven p.m. six nights a week, yet finds time to train between ten and twelve hours a week. "I have a coach who gives me my program, and I plan my week around it. I have backup safety plans. If I miss a ride, I can do it at home on the trainer after work." Yes, after leaving the restaurant at eleven p.m., he'll do a ninety-minute ride on a stationary bike. Some nights, he says, he'll think about missing a workout. "Like last night, I sat on the couch, fell asleep, then woke up and thought, 'I'm going to skip it.' But I got on the bike."

His dedication has paid off. "I do really well on the masters' level, which is riders over thirty years old, and I was state champion in California in all three of my events in 2010. I went to masters' nationals, and got a third place and a fifth place."

As he's reeling off his accomplishments—and I should say he wasn't bragging, just making sure I understood this wasn't some random thing he was doing in his practically nonexistent free time—his wife, Karen, is nodding along. She's more like most people I know: well-intentioned about exercise, but prey to the clock. "Something happens—you move or you open another restaurant, and it's difficult to maintain regular exercise," she says. Or, as happened to her just weeks after we met, you have another baby. But Quinn adds that Karen is actually good at fitting it all in somehow. "Before this pregnancy, she'd go to the gym and do an hour on the treadmill," he says. "Which seems crazy to me."

Lesson 72: They enlist an ally

Nancy Silverton is not a believer in hard-core workouts. "I play tennis—poorly—once a week," she says in a way that makes me believe her game isn't that poor. But she does start each day with an hour of exercise, usually under the watch of a trainer. "I train outside, because I don't like the gym. So we walk in the neighborhood with weights. I do push-ups against somebody's wall, and tie weight-resistant bands against somebody's fence. That's as much exercise as I can tolerate, but it's an important part of my day. I feel I've done a little bit of something."

If having a trainer once in a while is accessible to you, it can be a great motivator. Sue Torres uses hers a little differently from Silverton—she wants to keep the intensity of her workouts high, and knows she won't do it alone. So she has a standing date with a personal trainer for weights, kickboxing, and boxing. "I've given him permission to hit me with a stick when I mess up," she says, and even though she laughs when she says it, after a moment I realize she's serious.

She explains further: "That's what I understand—old-school. If I don't do a push-up right, he says, 'Do it again.' He won't hurt me, but he keeps me in line." You may not want such tough love. Her coach's method speaks to Torres, who, as a kid, toughed it out as the only girl on a boys' baseball team, after nagging her mom to play. Having to keep up with the boys would later serve her well in male-dominated kitchens. It also fired up her athletic side. While she no longer plays team sports, that kind of physicality remains integral to her life. "It's good to keep strong. I'm pretty fortunate in that I can eat whatever I want—and believe me, I eat an obscene amount of butter on bread. But I love it, and I work hard, so it's okay. It hasn't caught up with me yet."

Mark McEwan keeps in line with help from his wife, who is as committed to working out and watching how they eat as he is. "We are very much on the same page, very regimented." They each use the same trainer (separately) three days a week. "It's boxing routines, jumping, weights—an hour of pure torture," he says. "But without that I'd have to cut back what I eat even more."

Note: Get the right trainer, which may mean trying out a few. The first one Art Smith reached out to, he recalls, "told me he was Miley Cyrus's trainer. I was like, 'Uh-uh, no. I've got more fat on my finger.'"

A good teacher at a gym class can be a motivator too (not to mention a way to avoid the expense of one-on-one support). "I can't lose weight if I don't exercise," says Alex Guarnaschelli. "I spin. I take spinning classes until I can't see."

Lesson 73: **They bend to stay strong**

Professional cooking is itself a workout. I once heard a chef describe his job as "being paid to do aerobics in a sauna." Several have found that incorporating yoga into their workouts is a fine antidote to the labor of a kitchen. "Standing up on your feet working for that many hours, that many years, you just want to feel good," says Colorado chef Lachlan Mackinnon-Patterson. Before he opened his own restaurant, Frasca Food and Wine, he was part of a heady, talented team of chefs that included Alinea's Grant Achatz and Sou'Wester's Eric Ziebold, working under Thomas Keller at the French Laundry. His physical memories of that time are still with him: "We worked an incredible amount, and would drink Jamba Juice, the biggest possible, because we were starving, dehydrated, and tired. But it was a beautiful time to work there. Thomas is one of the great mentors. It was crazy energy."

These days Mackinnon-Patterson is the boss, and he isn't running crazed through his day, sucking on a sugary juice. But many of the physical demands of the job remain. "Yoga has changed my ability to continue doing it. I was someone who would come home from work and roll around on the floor or rub up against the wall like a bear." A visit from his friend Philadelphia chef Marc Vetri provided a better alternative. "He said yoga will change the way you feel, so I gave it a try. Oh, my God, I never felt that good."

Now that yoga is the core of his routine, which also includes biking to work, he says, "My back doesn't hurt. It became like getting dressed each day—I go all the time. I'm more calm and patient with my employees. Not because of any meditation, but you just take a breath and relax. It makes a difference. That and stretching the stiff joints and muscles have turned my life into a different kind of beauty."

Yoga does have a way of seeping out of that hour-long class and into other aspects of your life. While I've certainly used a lengthy run as justification for a big bowl of pasta followed by gelato, I don't think I've ever left a yoga studio with unhealthy cravings. Maybe I'm just highly suggestible, but I'm always in the mood for sweet potatoes, nutty brown rice, and green tea after yoga.

Rick Bayless is also a yoga devotee, though one who discovered his yoga-jock side only as an adult. "I came from a family of very athletic people who told me I was not athletic—and I believed them. From about second grade on, I never played a sport, because I was told I would not excel at it. Meanwhile, my brother was this star athlete," says Bayless, whose older brother, Skip, became an ESPN sportscaster.

"But I discovered when I was about forty I had potential. I was feeling lethargic, heavy—I'd gained some weight," recalls Bayless. "I just wanted to start moving, and I had a friend who was teaching yoga. She said, 'You'd love it; come over.' I did love the way it felt to move, to stretch. I started going to classes and there were all these postures I wanted to do, but I didn't have the strength to do them. So being the kind of guy I am, I didn't want to do yoga for ten more years to gain that strength. So I decided to go to a gym . . . but of course I was too embarrassed to go to a gym." So Bayless invested in some home weights, to build strength. "I still do three days of yoga and three days of weight training and cardio. I'm in the best shape of my life."

Like virtually everyone else who shared their fitness stories, Bayless found benefits that went beyond counteracting calories.

"The workout is my antidote to the pressured lifestyle. When people say, 'I'm too tired to go to the gym today; I think I'll blow it off,' I'm completely the opposite—I will be tired if I *don't* get to the gym. If I don't want to feel heavy and weighed down by the stresses of the day, I have to get to the gym; it's what gives me energy and releases stress."

Melissa Perello does yoga too, but the San Francisco chef says she can get a fine workout walking with her dog, Dingo. She is, like several of her colleagues, more of an exercise dabbler. When things get busy, she lets the workout slide a bit. But when she can, she says, "I try to ride my bike. I snowboard. I really like camping and hiking, just myself and my dog. I like being outside."

Yoga is one part of Cat Cora's weekly regimen, which might include cycling, climbing, hiking, swimming, or cardio and weights at the gym. Before becoming a chef, Cora earned a degree in exercise physiology. But she hasn't always been fighting-lean. "I was chubby in high school and gained the freshman fifteen in college. I wasn't eating right, and I wasn't exercising at all," she says. "If I stopped exercising and I ate anything I want, I could easily put weight on." She includes yoga and meditation in her training, because "both the active, outward things and the more inward things help balance my life with my crazy career and raising kids."

Ming Tsai has had a yoga practice for more than twenty years. A few times a week he takes a "hot yoga" class that, he says, "saves me. You sweat; you get all your toxins out. All chefs have toxins," he reports with authority. "But it's more than just physical; it really helps mentally too. You can't be thinking about work when you're on one foot with your other foot behind your head."

Lesson 74: **Eric Ripert hates exercise**

If none of the above speaks to you, you might be a four-star French chef. "I don't exercise at all. I hate exercising," insists Eric Ripert. He's six feet tall, and lean enough that Tom Colicchio wanted me to find out what his friend's secret is.

Ripert never goes to a gym or runs or any of that. What he does do, however, is make his morning commute a worthy substitute. Every day he walks from his Upper East Side home, through Central Park, to work on the west side of Midtown. The route is only about two miles, and takes him roughly forty minutes, so this isn't race-walking. But what's important to note about Ripert's routine is that when he says he does it every day, he doesn't mean every day the weather permits, or every day that he isn't in a big rush. He does it *every day.* "Even with a blizzard, or rain, or it's a hundred and twenty degrees outside, I do it."

Need proof? On a January morning when it was (I checked) ten degrees outside, and below zero with the wind chill factored in, Ripert was on his daily walk, posting online pictures of the icy road as he went. In his caption he's transposed letters in "Bernardin," so I imagine he was typing on his phone with gloves on. That's dedication. This is what it is to have a daily routine. It means every day. Really every day. Or as another chef put it, "I eat every day, right?"

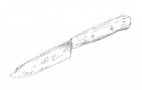

Art Smith's Chicken and Dumplings

This recipe originates with Art's mother, Addie Mae, whose dumplings are similar to flat, wide pappardelle noodles. Start with a good chicken and you will have broth that is fragrant and wonderful—if you can plan ahead a bit, cool the broth in the refrigerator for a few hours or overnight; this will make it easier to skim the fat off the top. Use other fresh herbs like chives or tarragon or savory in addition to (or instead of) the parsley, if you like.

serves 6

One 3- to 3½-pound chicken, cut into 8 pieces
1 medium onion, quartered
2 celery ribs, chopped
2 carrots, chopped
2 quarts water
Salt
Freshly ground black pepper

FOR THE DUMPLINGS:
1½ cups all-purpose flour
Salt
½ cup + 1 tablespoon water
1 tablespoon canola oil
2 tablespoons chopped fresh parsley

1. Place the chicken, onion, celery and carrots in a 5-quart Dutch oven or covered casserole and add the water, ½ teaspoon of salt, and ¼ teaspoon of pepper. Over high heat, bring to a boil. Reduce the heat to low and cover tightly.

Simmer, occasionally skimming off any foam that rises to the surface, until the chicken is tender, about 50 minutes.

2. Using tongs, transfer the chicken to a platter (keep the vegetables and broth simmering). When the chicken is cool enough to handle, remove the skin and cut the meat into bite-size pieces.

3. Meanwhile, increase the heat under the broth to high and cook until the liquid is reduced to about 6 cups. (If you're in a hurry, strain the broth, and return 6 cups of broth and the vegetables to the pot, reserving the rest for another use.) Skim off the fat from the surface and stir the chicken meat into the pot. Season to taste with salt and pepper.

4. While the soup is cooking, make the dumplings: Place the flour, salt, and oil in a medium bowl and gradually stir in the water to make a stiff dough. Turn out onto a lightly floured surface and knead briefly. Roll dough out to ¼ inch thick.

5. Using a sharp knife, cut the dough into strips that are about 1 inch by 2½ inches. Place on a plate in the freezer until ready to drop into the soup. Once the broth has reduced, slide the strips into the soup, without crowding them. Cover tightly and reduce heat to low. Simmer until the dumplings are cooked through and tender, about 10 minutes. Sprinkle with parsley, and serve the soup ladled into bowls.

Adapted from *Back to the Table: The Reunion of Food and Family* by Art Smith. Hyperion, 2001.

Joe Bastianich's White Bean Stew with Swiss Chard and Tomatoes

Because he's still a wine guy, I asked Joe what wine to pair with a vegetarian dish like this. His answer: a crisp Friulano.

serves 4 as a side dish

- 2 pounds Swiss chard, large stems discarded and leaves cut crosswise into 2-inch strips
- ¼ cup extra-virgin olive oil
- 3 garlic cloves, thinly sliced
- ¼ teaspoon crushed red pepper
- 1 cup canned tomatoes, chopped
- 16-ounce can cannellini beans, drained and rinsed
- Salt

1. Bring a saucepan of water to a boil. Add the chard and reduce the heat to medium and simmer until tender, about 8 minutes. Drain the greens and gently press out excess water.

2. In the same saucepan, warm the oil over medium heat. Add the garlic and crushed red pepper and cook until the garlic is golden, 1 minute. Add the tomatoes and bring to a boil. Add the beans and simmer for 3 minutes. Add the chard and simmer until the flavors meld, about 5 minutes. Season with salt to taste and serve.

Adapted from Joe Bastianich.

BEHIND THE LESSONS:

Rick Moonen's Paper Route to the Kitchen

Rick Moonen remembers being a really active boy who loved handball and gymnastics in school. "That was fun. Me against the world, running, jumping. And I always had a bicycle." The fourth of seven kids who lived with Mom, Dad, and Grandma in Flushing, Queens, Moonen describes a childhood that doesn't really exist anymore in New York City: one where there were so many siblings that you were, he says, "pretty much on your own," and an enterprising boy of ten could have a paper route that took him around the neighborhood and into the halls of strangers' apartment buildings without peril.

Besides giving him pocket money, the paper route offered him an early food education. "People grew fruit in their yards, and I knew where every fruit tree was: pears, sour cherries. It was awesome. I'd climb the trees, eat the fruit." He was responsible for delivering the afternoon papers to three apartment buildings in an enclave of mostly Italian, Greek, Jewish, Irish, and German families: "Take the elevator up to the top, and go down the stairs dropping off papers. On Friday night you had to go collect, and those hallways—the smells that would come out! Those dinners! I smelled fish cooking; it was really attractive to me. I'd never smelled lamb—my mother wasn't allowed to cook it, because my father said it made him sick to his stomach."

Moonen's father was Dutch, his mother German-Irish.

His dad had been, he says, "a spy for the government, taking pictures of what the Nazis were doing," and Mom was a nurse. When she came home from work, she cooked—you had to with seven kids. "She was the one-pot wonder, with that big cast-iron pot. Sloppy joes or Swedish meatballs—I loved those. Pot roast. Ham. Friday we had fish, and she would broil the shit out of it," he says with a laugh. Mom couldn't have known that he would grow up to be a master of fish cookery (with some notable dishes barely touching a flame).

"But no lamb, because my father came over on a boat. It was rough. Everybody got sick, including the crew. When you get that sick, they give you mutton tea, which is mutton boiled to a consommé. Mutton is very fatty and has a distinctive lamb stink to it, and for the rest of your life you don't want to smell that. So I never knew what lamb was, until I met the Greeks and discovered, 'This is awesome!'

"My next-door neighbor was an Italian with a butcher shop. I got to watch bones being ripped apart; I was intrigued—the smell of meat, sawdust on the floor. I was getting an education, and I was so curious. I ended up in the kitchen with my mother, because I was so active, I'd take the TV apart with a screwdriver if she didn't have me in the kitchen. I'd watch *The Galloping Gourmet* on TV. Graham Kerr—what a pisser. I loved it! Down the block from me was a couple named the Bontempis, who had a TV cooking show and lived in a gorgeous house. They would throw out the scripts and I'd pick them up from the garbage. They were in boxes," he hastens to add. "It wasn't like I was picking through banana peels."

From these beginnings, a chef. Moonen garnered notice at the Water Club, and then after six years jumped to

Oceana, where he earned three stars from the *New York Times*. "Boom! My life changes: You're the fish guy," he says. "Typecasting." But he embraced the role and, still that enterprising kid inside, used it to voice concern about using seafood responsibly. It's an issue that is much discussed now, but was barely on anyone's radar at the time. In 1998 he signed on as a spokesman for the national "Give Swordfish a Break" campaign.

Eventually Moonen became a TV chef too. Full circle. But he says, "I don't have a romance with myself. I watch a show once to make sure I didn't look like a jerk." He claims not to care how he looks, although he does want to stay fit. Exercise, he says, "makes me a better boss, a better businessman." But the gymnastics he did as a teen, he says, had "screwed up my back nice. Then long hours in the kitchen didn't help." To his surprise, he found the best thing for him was Pilates, which he took up at the urging of a customer in Las Vegas, a Pilates instructor. "So now I do Pilates. And I still ride my bicycle. I put on my headphones and I'm in my own world."

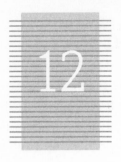

EAT AROUND
THE WORLD

CHEFS ARE TRAVELERS. And travelers, when they're lucky, can sometimes experience the most wonderful paradox: They treat themselves because they are on vacation, and yet often find they haven't gained a pound. Walking the monuments of Rome apparently more than offsets the gelato you consume there. Same with croissants in Paris. (Would that it were so for pizza in New York.)

But eating on the road also has its challenges, and unfortunately not every time we pack our bags do we have the luxury of being tourists. There are business trips with little in ambulatory sightseeing. There are long flights plagued by boredom eating and bad meals. There are layovers with nothing but fast-food outlets in the airport. "It's fascinating to me that we've come so far in the world, but transit dining is still in 1982," observes Marcus Samuelsson, who travels frequently to Europe, Asia, Africa, and around the States. Being stuck interminably in a terminal with no good food is something with which he struggles. "As a chef, I spend a lot of time in the airport. It's the hardest thing in the world."

So here several chefs discuss two important points: One, how to avoid the worst offenses that airports, hotels, and jet lag inflict on our otherwise healthy habits; and two, how to embrace the best aspects of travel, from enjoying authentic ethnic meals to bringing home inspiration for eating well after you return.

Lesson 75: Smart chefs have a flight plan

"I try to eat before I go to the airport," says Samuelsson. By doing so, he can usually ignore the poor offerings in most terminals. But when a three-hour flight turns into double that in delays, even he is not immune from eating the garbage on offer beyond the security checkpoint. "Sometimes I just punk out and have to do it. I don't feel good about it after. I wish I could say I never do, but I don't." His alternative plan: "Sometimes I look at it as an opportunity to take my day of fasting."

If there is someone who travels farther and more often than Alain Ducasse, I don't know who he is. The multiple Michelin three-star chef has restaurants and hotels bearing his name in New York, Las Vegas, Tokyo, Hong Kong, Tuscany, and, of course, in Paris and his adopted home of Monaco. When I met him in December 2010, he was making plans for a new restaurant in St. Petersburg, Russia. "I am never more than a week without getting on a plane," he tells me. We met at the launch of a Ducasse iPad app, designed for the world traveler to keep straight all the locales in the chef's global empire.

This much travel can strain one's diet, exposing the traveler to a flying circus of bad airplane meals. (I don't care what sort of superior, premium, ultra-first-class you fly; it's still reheated in foil.) But Ducasse appears to have it all in hand. Like Samuelsson, he says, "I eat before I get to the airport." But never what's served at thirty-five thousand feet. If he gets hungry midflight, his wife has usually packed him "very healthy" snacks, he says, such as vegetables or a homemade muesli. No sweets. "She doesn't think I need dessert." He also feels that eating a meal with plenty of protein and drinking lots of water when you land at your destination help put you back on schedule.

Wolfgang Puck is another peripatetic chef, on the road about two hundred days a year. "For me, the airplane is the best way to diet," he jokes. "I never eat on the plane." This usually comes as a relief to flight attendants who recognize Puck and feel timid about serving him the pod meals they sling at the rest of us. "I say, 'It's fine; I'm on a diet.'" Otherwise, he says, he eats a little at home before he takes off (or sometimes at the airport— he does sell a lot of pizzas there) and then "just go to sleep."

Here's another Puck suggestion for you to try someday, should you also find yourself the guest on the private plane of a casino magnate. "I just flew back to Los Angeles from Singapore with Sheldon Adelson on his plane, so I brought some steak, and I grilled steaks in the kitchen—they have a kitchen on the plane," reports Puck. "We had a salad with it. Everybody loved it! That's the only way to travel."

Lesson 76: When they arrive, smart chefs eat like locals

Depending on where your travels take you, eating like a native can keep your weight in check. "In France, in Italy, in parts of

China, you don't find heavy people, because they have great food all the time," notes Rick Bayless. "They eat, typically, with a little bit more patience. They don't have to gobble food thinking they are never going to get another great meal—they are!" It's an optimistic way of looking at the world, and pretty easy to subscribe to, even after you come home. There will be other good meals—don't treat each one as if it is your plate-licking last.

Being far from home can feed you such novel sensory feasts that you may find that you don't miss the worst parts of the standard American diet. Near the start of her career, Alex Guarnaschelli lived in Paris, where she worked for Guy Savoy. She was eating plenty, but also eating better than she had before. In France, she recalls, "My diet had next to no processed food in it. I love processed food like any American—I don't want you to write, 'She never eats Doritos,' because I do. But there, I naturally gravitated to a diet with a lot less processed food. And I just didn't eat as much—I was fed a lot by the sensory experiences of going to the market. I was in another culture, and I ate the way they did. We ate smaller portions, and the stuff I ate was *so good*. I ate cheese that would make anybody cry. There were cheeses that I ate in the south of France that weren't available in Paris. Or cheeses in Paris that weren't available in other regions. Sometimes eating something that doesn't taste like anything you've eaten before has a different effect in feeding you. If you're an emotional eater like I am, then maybe your emotions are fed in a different way and maybe you eat less. I think that is some of what happened. I'm simplifying it, but I think a different environment, different culture, different language, different foods can definitely change the way you eat, and I think in this case it was for the better."

Lesson 77: **They eat authentic cuisines**

If you have the good fortune to travel abroad to a country with a great food lineage, don't waste a moment eating in a hotel with an American-style breakfast buffet. Simpson Wong, raised in Malaysia but living in New York since 1988, has traveled widely: to Hong Kong, India, Southeast Asia, Europe, and elsewhere. (He was so determined to keep one Paris reservation, he asked his cardiologist for permission to travel days after a heart attack; permission denied.) He has one rule: "I never eat the breakfast in a hotel. Hotel breakfast is all sausage and bacon and eggs—it's not my cup of tea," he says. Instead, "I go to the market, and walk around and eat whatever they have to offer. I go see the old ladies selling vegetables—it's a fun thing for me. I'm not interested in toast with butter."

Another suggestion: Seek out local dining options while you do your morning workout, as Nate Appleman does. While running, "I see different parts of cities. I'll just get lost. In Tokyo I was literally lost—I mean to the point where I was showing people my hotel room key and saying, 'Where is this?' That's a good way to travel."

Often the indigenous cuisine is generally healthier before being adapted to foreign palates. "U.S. Chinese food is not Chinese food," says Wong. "If you're eating General Tso's chicken, you're actually eating a McNugget. They take meat, coat it in a batter, and deep-fry it and serve it with a molasses-laden sauce." He notes some other differences: "The English language says, 'Eat soup'; the Chinese language says, 'Drink soup.' Real wonton soup is a chicken broth, a consommé with something to garnish it. In the West, the entire thing is wonton."

At the same time, it's wise to bring along your good judgment. Just because you're eating in a land that is generally known for healthy food doesn't mean everything can be consumed with abandon. "Look at what it is," says Susur Lee, who offers this example: "There's a Beijing dish that is fish 'swimming' in oil. It's not what Western people are used to." If you are going for that delicacy, make sure you enjoy it as the locals do, with chopsticks, tapping off excess oil. "If you eat it with a fork, you'll get all the oil." In Italy you don't need to have antipasto, pasta, a *secondo*, and dessert at every dinner simply because it is there. Sometimes when in Rome, you should still eat to your own hunger cues.

Once you've enjoyed real versions of great cuisines, you can seek them out when you return home. When we came back from a family vacation in China, my husband and I were hardly experts (that would take decades). But we knew enough to now look for the best examples in New York of the spicy dishes we had enjoyed in Chengdu.

If you live in a good-size American city, you don't need to leave town to enjoy "foreign" dining adventures on a regular basis. One morning, I accidentally found myself in a new corner of Brooklyn at a Russian coffee shop, which seemed to have its roots in both St. Petersburg and Seattle, with custom-brewed coffee and Russian specialties. (If you must know why I was there: My son forgot his gym shoes and I was passing time waiting for a shoe store to open somewhere near Cobble Hill—which sounds like it should have shoes everywhere, but doesn't.) The coffee shop had kasha and onions on the menu—something I can't get at any of my usual bruncheries just thirty minutes over the river in Manhattan. A great breakfast with whole grains and Soviet-era attitude from the staff—no passport needed.

Lesson 78: They enjoy some local specialties only on location

Raised in Mississippi, Cat Cora has long lived in California, and now exemplifies the best of that state's healthy lifestyle. At home, family dinner is often outdoors around the grill: fish, chicken, vegetables, and stone fruit for dessert. But she hasn't forsaken her favorite Southern specialties—fried chicken, biscuits, buttery grits. "I do crave that every once in a while," she says. "When I go home, I'll definitely stop for a really great biscuit or a big bowl of grits."

Rather than making them a regular part of her life in the West, she limits them to visits to Mississippi. "It's food you can't eat every day," says Cora. "I mean, a lot of people do, but that's why we have a lot of obesity in the South." Not to pick on the South, of course. California, too, has its once-in-a-while indulgences. Locals who have a problem with In-N-Out Burger addiction should probably leave those to visitors.

Travel can give you a pass to indulge in a way you would not at home. I will never go to New Orleans and not eat a beignet at Café Du Monde; for that matter I'll never go to Disneyland and not queue up for the seriously substandard "New Orleans fritter" they sell next to the Haunted Mansion—environment is everything, and sugared dough fried in oil and nostalgia is hard to pass up. Do I ever eat fried dough at home? No, never.

As long as this sort of situational eating is an anomaly, it shouldn't be a problem. It all depends on where you're going and for how long. During his years running two eponymous hotel restaurants in Las Vegas, Alex Stratta would watch how people ate, and saw that they were not really there for spa cuisine. "I had vegan dishes," which guests rarely ordered, he says. "People come to Vegas to get debauched for two days and go home. You don't see as many people in the gym as in the nightclub."

Lesson 79: **They take home inspiration**

Chefs travel as a matter of professional education—and because it's fun. Just before we met up, Marcus Samuelsson had been in Texas as part of an ongoing exploration of American barbecue. "Part of being a chef is being completely humble about what you don't know. If you're in any creative field and take the opportunity to learn, you have an amazing opportunity to become really good."

"I did a lot of traveling to learn food," says Michelle Bernstein. "My favorite growing up was always fish and seafood. I lived in the south of France for a while. In Marseilles I learned a proper bouillabaisse. Then I went to Peru for a while to learn the ceviches and anticuchos and the beautiful tiraditos and all that good stuff. Then, obviously, I lived with what my mother taught me in the kitchen. My cooking is kind of a big mishmosh of all that."

"Eating is a good education, if you have the mind of a cook," says Andrea Reusing. Sometimes when she finds herself facing an uninspired menu, she often thinks, *This person just needs to travel! Travel, or read the cookbooks that can offer some of the same thing.*

Like chefs, laypeople can learn something about the preparation of the foreign or regional cuisines we love, and incorporate new ideas into our home cooking for lighter and more flavorful dishes. While in Yangshuo, China, I took a cooking class at a school that overlooked the Li River. For me, simply learning the proper way to heat and add food to a wok with the right amount of oil was worth the whole journey.

You needn't venture so far—I do only rarely. A summer vacation in Maine found me, quite accidentally, on a guided mushroom walk. I thought the only thing I might come away with was a good anecdote about tromping around with an amateur mycologist. Instead, I learned a lot. (The major takeaway: The most adorable mushrooms can destroy your central nervous system faster than the virus that killed off Gwyneth Paltrow in *Contagion*.) Further, I was prompted to come home and cook with mushrooms I often overlook in the market: chanterelles (did you know there are several wild varieties, not all edible?), lobster mushrooms (actually two fungi—one living off the other), and black trumpets (delicious, but not without indelicate repercussions if consumed in excess; eat them with pasta, not a plateful on their own). There's a lot more to know about mushrooms, but that was just enough information on a memorably odd day to move me to experiment with a whole category of food I hadn't much considered before. It's a souvenir I hadn't expected to bring home.

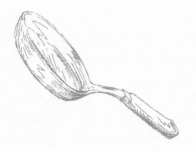

Simpson Wong's Black Bass with Lemongrass Salad

serves 4 as a main course

FOR THE SALAD:

- ½ cup lemongrass, thinly sliced and separated into rings
- ½ cup celery, tough stringy parts removed with a vegetable peeler, and thinly sliced on the diagonal
- ⅓ cup chopped cilantro
- ⅓ cup thinly sliced scallions
- ½ cup diced red bell pepper
- 1 tablespoon minced shallots
- 1 small garlic clove, minced
- ⅓ cup extra-virgin olive oil
- 1 tablespoon of coconut vinegar*
- 2 teaspoons salt
- 1½ teaspoons sugar
- ¼ teaspoon chili flakes
- 1 tablespoon fresh lime juice*

FOR THE FISH:

- 4 to 5 ounces black sea bass fillets
- Salt and freshly ground pepper
- 2 tablespoons olive oil

1. Toss all the salad ingredients in a large bowl so that the vegetables are coated with dressing.

2. Season bass fillets with salt and pepper.

3. Warm the olive oil in a large nonstick pan over medium heat. Place the bass fillets skin-side down. Press the top of each fillet lightly with a spatula to prevent it from curling up. Cook the fish until the skin is crispy, about 5 minutes. Turn the fillets over and cook for another 2 minutes.

4. Place each fillet on a plate. Divide the lemongrass salad evenly and place on the top of the fillet. Serve immediately.

*Coconut vinegar has a tartness and sharpness that's different from other vinegars. You can substitute rice wine vinegar or white balsamic, but both tend to be sweeter. If using these, add another tablespoon of lime juice.

Adapted from Simpson Wong.

BEHIND THE LESSONS:

Andrea Reusing's Tea-smoked Chicken

I first saw the recipe for Andrea Reusing's tea-smoked chicken in *Food & Wine* magazine. Intrigued by the description of the unusual flavors and tender results of smoking, then roasting, I read it through—from cooking and cooling the ten-ingredient brine to fashioning a smoker on my stovetop—and promptly decided this was a dish best enjoyed in the restaurant that serves it. I might attempt it today, but back then I lacked the confidence. It's a real chef's recipe.

Fortunately, I eventually did get to Reusing's lovely Chapel Hill restaurant, Lantern, for a dinner with our friends Steven and Jim, who are lucky enough to call themselves regulars there. I got to enjoy the juicy, smoky chicken that was, as described, fragrant with star anise and toasty tea.

Reusing didn't start her career with a culinary school degree. She was working for a public-policy consultant in New York when she moved with her future husband, a musician, to North Carolina. "I'd line-cooked when I was in college. When I moved, I wanted to get involved in food, but I didn't know how exactly. So I started an illegal home-catering operation. Then I was hired to open a restaurant for people who had never opened a restaurant before. I taught myself by reading and eating out."

The small wine-focused restaurant was a success. But, tired of having bosses, Reusing eventually ventured out on her own, with a modern pan-Asian-influenced restaurant, though by that point she had yet to travel anywhere in Asia. "When I was catering, people responded to the Asian food I made. There weren't a lot of Asian restaurants in the area," she recalls. "So it was something I could do well and it filled a need in the community. People were still opening expense-account American restaurants, and I felt like that market was a little crowded. Initially my younger brother was my partner. We were both in the kitchen, and had a fun, tumultuous couple of years. Then he left, so we're still friends."

When she first opened, she worked without recipes. But after having two babies, she learned to delegate and is now meticulous about recipe writing. The tea-smoked chicken has been on the menu since day one. A lot of people have tried it and loved it.

One person who hasn't tasted it happens to be married to the chef. Why? "He's punishing me," Reusing explains, only half joking. Her husband hasn't tasted most of the dishes on her inventive menu, because he doesn't eat anything with feet (he's a vegetarian who sometimes eats fish). She blames his conversion on "a girlfriend he had when he was seventeen, who was a vegetarian." The irony (and now Reusing is really fake-fuming . . .) is "now she comes into my restaurant and orders lamb! I'm sorry; I am *not* serving you lamb—you ruined my life! My husband won't even eat stock!"

So at home with her family, Reusing cooks mostly meat-free (the kids seem to be taking after their dad). She makes beans, soups, egg dishes, pastas, salads. "Very simple things." She adds, "I never cook Asian food at home. It seems like too much work."

It can be, sure. But that doesn't mean that we won't sometimes try. Because it may be a while until I'm back in North Carolina, and I think I still have that chicken recipe somewhere.

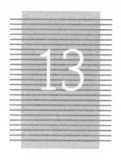

EAT AFTER EATING
FOR TWO

"As a chef, I did justice to my kind by gaining seventy-five pounds when I was pregnant," says a reliably unabashed Alex Guarnaschelli. "I really enjoyed that. It was a unique metabolic experience."

Oh, I know just what she means. With the exception of some heartburn at the five-month mark, my forty-one weeks of pregnancy were consistently among the best of my eating life. I did miss wine and raw fish. But I more than compensated with weekly post-prenatal yoga class visits to the City Bakery on Eighteenth Street for pretzel croissants and cups of hot cocoa. (The supersecret recipe, best I can tell, is heavy cream, dark chocolate, and a double chin.)

I wanted to know how mom-chefs eat, and I began by comparing notes with several about their pregnancies and how they ate and worked out during and after. Cat Cora kept up her ambitious routine, but modified the intensity. "I was still doing exercise every day, but I was walking or something low-impact. I don't know how women jog when they're pregnant; I really don't." That made me feel better, knowing a jock like Cora is also scratching her head over that one.

Though I initially began thinking only about new moms and their baby weight, eating after you become a parent involves much more than trying to drop those hanging-on pounds. All of a sudden there's another eater in the household. That new eater may do fine on only breast milk for a long while, but eventually she wants food—even before they have words, children have strong opinions about food, and they will have a huge impact on the home menu. Will you insist they eat what you're eating, prepare separate adult and kids' meals, or find yourself matching your kid one-to-one on peanut-butter-and-jelly-sandwich consumption? And how do smart chefs manage to eat right in the face of a punishing lack of time and sleep?

In this chapter, you will hear how some mom-chefs got back in prebaby shape. But you'll also hear from moms and dads about how the newest member of the family changed how they eat, and how they adapted. If you aren't much of a home cook, it might please you to know that, until they become parents, neither are many restaurant chefs. When her daughter was about three and a half, Guarnaschelli told me, "This past year has been the most home cooking I've ever done. I want my daughter to see an example of a parent who cooks. There's a certain way that you show love when you cook for someone, and I want her to feel loved in that way. I don't do it because I'm a chef. I do it because I want her to know I love her in that way."

Some people may find this controversial—the idea of showing love through cooking. I don't. The feeling that comes when someone you love unconditionally is happily eating food you've prepared is without comparison.

Lesson 80: Smart chefs don't stress about losing all the baby weight right away

Can we agree to stop reading interviews with actresses who claim to have lost all their pregnancy weight solely by nursing their infants or running the three steps it takes to catch a toddler? "Everyone says, 'You're breast-feeding—the weight falls right off you!' But I found that as long as I was breast-feeding, I held on to weight and ate a ton. It's the best time to eat!" says Andrea Reusing, who has a son and a daughter. "I had *great* eating experiences then. I'd have peanut butter with really good jam and bread and hot chocolate with whipped cream. I didn't lose all the weight until I stopped breast-feeding." Me too. I had this idea that making milk meant drinking milk (not a bad idea), and that drinking milk meant always eating Oreos (not a sane idea).

Karen Hatfield also took it pretty easy after the birth of her first child. "I lost twenty pounds immediately, then the other fifteen in six months. That's my thing: I'm not going to go in the gym and kill myself to get the abs I had when I was twenty. It's important to me to be slim, to be at an appropriate weight, but I'm not too hard on myself, and I think that's a good thing. Also, I figured, 'If you're going to have another kid, you're not going to work to get the dream body. I'll get the trainer after the second one.'"

That would be soon. "Do you know how to deliver a baby?" Quinn Hatfield asks me by way of greeting when I enter the restaurant he runs with his, at that time, very pregnant wife. She is something of a marvel, nearing forty weeks with their second child and still at Hatfield's every day, making pastry and managing the restaurant. I arrive in the afternoon, well before they open for dinner, and the place has a sort of sterile hush that makes me consider whether, with judicious use of the dish sanitizer, we could deliver the baby if we absolutely had to.

"With the last baby, Karen worked Saturday, we were closed on Sunday, she had the baby Monday, and she was back to work on Friday," says Quinn in both admiration and disbelief. Says Karen: "We're youngish, trying to run a restaurant, maybe open another one. All these things take time and commitment, and just being there." So here she is, prioritizing. "Maybe after the second baby I'll get a trainer," she muses.

"I thought I was going to train you!" says Quinn, smiling at his wife.

Taking in the dining room with her eyes, she says to him, "Isn't this enough?" She turns to me for confirmation: "Is there anything worse than your husband training you post-baby? Biggest nightmare!"

Alex Guarnaschelli had great success at taking off nearly all the weight she put on with her daughter, but says, "I'm still in the process of trying to lose my baby weight—I want to be very clear about that. I don't want to be portrayed as anything but an ever-struggling human." With exercise, and some decisive changes to her diet, she steadily lost about sixty pounds. "I took out the high-ticket items. I'm a carnivore at heart, so I eliminated red meat. And salad dressing."

I find the no-dressing tack a hard-core choice. Personally, I don't like the scrape and squeak of lettuce without at least a little slick of oil; I need dressing to marry the leaves to the other elements in the salad, like members of a band wearing the same uniform, Sgt. Pepper style.

But I admire Alex's ability to go to the dry-salad place and even enjoy it. She explains, "I love greens. You have got to find your weird stuff that makes you laugh to yourself in the kitchen, your nutty little thing that works. I'm not telling anybody how to live. *For me*, I'm going to eliminate salad dressing and red meat and use my calories elsewhere and have some steamed fish so I can eat a little more food and feel satiated. I can't handle being on a diet and not feeling satiated. Because that is how I'll quickly go off the diet: day four of 'I'm really hungry all the time.'"

Lesson 81: They eat with their kids

Experts from nutritionists to sociologists have validated the benefits to children of eating at least some meals together as a family. But I think it serves all of us well. While we're encouraging our kids to eat their vegetables, chances are we are setting an example by eating them too. But there's a tendency among schedule-challenged parents to feed their kids well at mealtimes, and later cobble something together for themselves.

Here's one small example of why dining should be a social activity from a person's earliest days. When their daughter first started eating solid foods, says Karen Hatfield, she and her husband treated her like their most precious customer ever. "Quinn made all her baby food, sourcing this amazing stuff from farms, all organic—red quinoa, different squashes. Fabulous." (You can do this too, by the way; there is almost nothing that can't be cooked soft and pureed for the toothless newcomer.) But with their ambitious schedules, they rarely slowed down to eat with her. Now, Karen continues, admitting something that is hard for her as a chef and mother: "She's not the best eater. We're trying to wait it out and not put too much pressure on so she doesn't rebel."

The pickiness concerned them enough to raise the question with their daughter's pediatrician. "The doctor said it might have something to do with the fact that we're never home at night," Karen says. "Kids are more likely to eat if there's a big dish put down on the family table and everybody's drawing from it. I thought it made sense, and it made me feel better. It's hard for me to eat at seven with her, but I've been trying to make us both dinner and sit down."

Like the Hatfields, you too probably encounter times (perhaps several days a week) when making and eating dinner together challenges you, and there's a temptation to sling some dinner in your children's general direction and, when they are in bed, to have a glass of wine and a knob of cheese yourself before collapsing. But by making a simple meal and sitting down with your kids—by feeding yourself as sensibly as you expect them to eat—you may end up helping yourself too. I've often thought if I ate half as well as I encourage my son to eat, I'd be so healthy that you could see me glowing from space. If I'm taking the time to prepare food for him, I would do well to sit down and eat some myself.

Two or three nights a week, Ming Tsai brings home a few raw ingredients from his restaurant, Blue Ginger, to get something fast on the table by six p.m. Most nights his wife, Polly, is in charge, though she is also hustling, says Tsai. "With two kids, picking up and dropping off from squash practice or karate class, you don't have all day to hang out and cook." Some nights, he says, "I have dinner with my family, and then I come back for service."

One of Andrea Reusing's best family dining tricks is to offer a predinner crudité: "I'll just put out a ton of vegetables before

I put any other food out, so they get their vegetables in them when they're most hungry. Then they can go to town on whatever else they want." Hint: This works on adults too.

Reusing also makes it easy on herself, preparing adaptable foods in bulk, and keeping staples on hand. "I make a batch of chickpeas or some bean a couple times a week, and use them different ways," she says. "Or sometimes we have egg dinners. I get the best eggs I can, from a farm." Breakfast for dinner is almost too easy—you get it to the table fast, and very young children are delighted by the idea of turning routine upside down.

There may be times when eating a full meal with your progeny is just not practical—maybe you're going out later and don't want to eat twice. Wolfgang Puck often makes it home, even briefly, for dinner with his boys. But he doesn't necessarily eat what he or his wife, Gelila, prepares for them. "I've eaten during the day, and I'm going to eat more afterward," says Puck, who usually returns to Spago for dinner service. "I will nibble a bit, but not really eat. It's an important time to all be together. Then I go back to work."

In a best-case scenario, having a kid in the house makes you eat better than you did before. "It makes you think about the four food groups. So we'll have more fruit salad, more vegetables," says Frasca chef Lachlan Mackinnon-Patterson, of cooking for his young daughter. Before he heads to work, Lachlan packs her lunch most days, which might be anything from some of his restaurant's leftover staff meal, to pasta salad, little meatballs, and raspberries "she sticks on her fingers."

He delights in that daddy stuff, but he never really stops being a chef, and chefs are constantly watching the plates to see whether they come back to the kitchen empty. "I'm always thinking about what's in her lunch, and I check when she comes home to see what she ate," he says. "If she doesn't eat it,

I wonder why and I call her teacher." I think he is joking about calling the teacher. But for chefs, and other parents, it is hard not to read your reviews. Kids can be tough food critics, and for most of us cooks, theirs are the only names in the reservation book for nearly two decades.

Lesson 82: They don't fall into the "kiddie food" trap

Just because you eat *with* a kid doesn't mean you should eat *like* a kid. With peanut butter and jelly in my refrigerator all the time, I sometimes have to make it invisible to myself, but doing so is surprisingly possible if there are plenty of other, more appropriate treats. A favorite Susur Lee snack: a sweet potato. Make extra next time you roast them. Nate Appleman says, "We always have nuts or dried fruit, cheese, or almond butter. I've actually grown to love graham crackers—they are a not-too-indulgent sweet."

If my son had his way we would eat some type of pasta most nights. If I ate pasta at every dinner, I imagine you would be able to roll me down Fifth Avenue like a giant croquet ball through the wicket of the Washington Square arch. One way to resolve that issue is to make a pasta side dish, rather than the sole element in a meal. I try not to do even that too often, and need to remind myself that couscous and orzo are, in fact, pasta, not grains, despite their attempts to deceive me with their tiny size and grainlike shape.

Unless you are planning to make multiple dinners every night (don't—home is not a restaurant!), a better way to bridge the kiddie-food/grown-up-food divide is to do what chefs do and introduce your kids to a variety of foods—and make them appealing to young palates—so you can get off the pasta train.

Cat Cora and her wife, Jennifer, cook the healthy dinners they want—grilled fish, chicken, vegetables—and have found that putting any of those things on a stick sells them to their four boys without a fuss. "The kids love it," she says. "We'll do a salmon skewer and romesco sauce [a Spanish sauce of nuts, garlic, olive oil, and peppers], or lamb with mint-yogurt sauce and pita bread."

Romesco sauce? Yes! First of all, it's pink, if you have the kind of child to whom that makes a difference. Who says kid food needs to be bland? "When I sautéed vegetables for my kids, I would add oyster sauce, or clear clam juice," says Susur Lee, father of three. "The umami sweetness is attractive to kids." Another tip: They might need vegetables prepped slightly differently from yours. "Dice them small for children," he adds.

"My kids like vegetables, as long as they are flavorful," says Ming Tsai. "I'll use a cast-iron pan to caramelize a bunch of garlic and sauté broccoli with vegetable stock, put some herbed panko on top of it, under the broiler for eight minutes. I take pride and love cooking for my family. They love good food and appreciate it, so it's fun to do."

Lesson 83: They cook with their kids

Getting kids into the kitchen is another way to get them excited about the kind of food you want to serve and eat. On Sunday, his day off, Tsai likes to cook with his boys. "We'll make dumplings, sushi, stir-fries, fried rice." Tsai prefers the nutrients, fiber, and flavor of brown rice, but knows that kids are more apt to go for white. His solution is to mix the two in fried rice, and his guys, he says, don't notice the difference.

Reusing, too, taps her offspring as mini sous chefs. "I like to make something with them that they get invested in but that doesn't create a lot of work," she says. "Like ricotta gnocchi. I make the gnocchi, and let them spoon them into the boiling water."

"Last night we made bread and onion soup," reports Nate Appleman of a Sunday evening spent cooking with his young son. I don't have statistics on this, but I feel safe in saying that the majority of American children are not clamoring for onion soup most nights. Could Oliver be sold on it? Yes, Appleman found, though it took two attempts. "I burned the onions because we were playing trains or something," he admits. "It was a big, black mess. I changed the pot and it worked out. We also did the Jim Lahey no-knead bread, which turned out great." (Lahey's much-reproduced method can be found at www.sullivanstreetbakery.com/recipes). Appleman shows me a photo of his son holding the loaf—the boy looks as proud as can be. Remember the rule about eating only really special bread? This would be that.

Lesson 84: Smart chefs don't sacrifice shared food experiences for their diets

Besides the convenience of cooking one meal for all, eating the same food has another benefit, and that is teaching kids that good food is good for everybody. Just because I'm watching how I eat, I don't want my son growing up to think that certain foods are okay for him, but not for Mommy or Daddy.

Some chefs agree with me. "There's enough advertising to make kids self-conscious" about food and diet and weight, says Marc Murphy, a dad of two. "If my kids want an ice-cream cone, even if I'm not that hungry, I'll get an ice-cream cone, because I don't want to be that parent who's like, 'Oh, I can't eat that!' We'll all have ice cream together. It's fun. You want to teach them to live and enjoy life."

While it can upset my own best intentions for the day, I do the same when I'm out with my son. We live in New York, where as we stroll up the avenue there is not only the siren call of the Mister Softee truck, but pizza by the slice to be had, soft pretzels with salt and mustard. We don't always stop for these treats, but to pass them by altogether would be sort of tragic. Honestly, if I were ever to become too careful an eater to enjoy a greasy slice from Ray's Pizza, I don't belong in this city. So I try to find a balance, for myself and for him, hoping that as he grows up he's able to make good choices on his own.

Rick Bayless feels like he has accomplished that. "My daughter is now going to college. Sometimes she eats good food, sometimes not. But what she's learned is to be aware when she's full. She'll say, 'This is superdelicious, but this is how much I can eat of it.' I think that will stand her in good stead for the rest of her life."

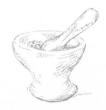

Cat Cora's Halibut "Gyros"

Traditional Greek gyros consist of lamb with tzatziki wrapped in pita. Cora retains the tzatziki (a garlicky yogurt sauce) in her version, which uses either grilled or baked fish. She recommends halibut, which is firm and holds up to being eaten by hand, gyros style—kids can assemble their own. But napkins are essential for all.

serves 4 to 6

FOR THE TZATZIKI:

- 1 cup Greek (strained) yogurt
- 2 tablespoons crumbled feta cheese
- 2 tablespoons extra-virgin olive oil
- 1 tablespoon fresh lemon juice
- 2 teaspoons finely chopped fresh mint
- 1 large garlic clove, minced
- 1 teaspoon kosher salt
- 1 medium cucumber, peeled

FOR THE HALIBUT:

- 2 tablespoons extra-virgin olive oil, plus more to sear the fish and to oil the baking dish
- 2 tablespoons fresh lime juice
- 1 teaspoon chili powder
- 1 tablespoon ground cumin
- 1 teaspoon cayenne pepper
- 1½ teaspoons sea salt
- ¼ teaspoon freshly ground pepper
- 1½ pounds center-cut halibut fillets, skin removed

FOR THE TOMATO SALAD:

5 Roma tomatoes, about 1¼ pounds

1 small red onion

½ cup kalamata olives, pitted and halved

1 tablespoon finely chopped fresh oregano

2 tablespoons parsley, roughly chopped

2 tablespoons extra-virgin olive oil

2 tablespoons fresh lime juice

Kosher salt and freshly ground pepper to taste

FOR SERVING:

1 head butter lettuce

1 head radicchio

Tzatziki

Pepperoncini, drained and sliced, optional

Sliced scallions, optional

1. Preheat a grill to medium-high or turn an oven to 350°F.

2. Make the tzatziki: In a medium bowl, combine all the ingredients except cucumber. Using a box grater, grate the cucumber directly over the yogurt mixture, rotating the cucumber and grating until all the flesh is used, stopping when you reach the seeds. Stir well, cover the bowl, and refrigerate for at least an hour, preferably overnight.

3. For the halibut: In a baking dish large enough to hold the fillets in a single layer, combine the 2 tablespoons olive oil, lime juice, chili powder, cumin, cayenne, salt, and pepper. Add the halibut and turn to coat thoroughly with the marinade. Let the fillets marinate for 10 minutes to absorb the flavors while you make the tomato salad.

4. For the tomato salad: In a medium bowl, mix the tomatoes, red onion, olives, oregano, parsley, olive oil, and lime juice. Season with salt and pepper to taste and mix well.

5. Cook the halibut: Remove the halibut fillets from the marinade. Brush the fillets with a little olive oil on each side before placing them on the grill. Cook the fillets until they start to turn opaque around the sides, about 3 to 5 minutes. Using a spatula, turn the fish carefully and grill on the other side until opaque throughout, about 3 to 5 minutes.

6. If you are baking the halibut, remove the fish from the marinade. Lightly oil the baking dish and place the halibut in a single layer. Bake in the preheated oven until firm to the touch and opaque throughout, about 15 minutes. When the fish is done, remove it from the oven and let it rest in the pan.

7. For serving: Remove the core from the lettuce and radicchio. Gently separate the lettuce leaves from one another. For extra-crisp lettuce cups, soak the lettuce leaves in very cold water for a few minutes. Remove them from the water and pat dry with paper towels. Make a cup by lining a whole lettuce leaf with a radicchio leaf (you can use 2 lettuce leaves if you prefer more lettuce with your gyros and to reduce the chance of leaks).

8. Flake a generous portion of fish into each of the lettuce cups. Top with the tomato salad, drizzle with the tzatziki, and garnish with pepperoncinis and scallions, if desired. Serve immediately.

Adapted from *Cooking from the Hip: Fast, Easy, Phenomenal Meals* by Cat Cora, with Ann Krueger Spivak. Houghton Mifflin Harcourt, 2007.

Naomi Pomeroy's Quinoa
with Summer Vegetables

This is a very adaptable recipe that Pomeroy makes at home for herself and her daughter. Use the vegetables you most like, or whatever you have on hand. Corn cut off the cob is a great addition. Make sure to rinse the quinoa well before cooking to avoid any bitterness. Even with that extra step, quinoa is among the fastest-cooking grains—a relief when you don't have time to wait for brown rice or others that take longer. It also has a fair amount of protein.

serves 4

½ head broccoli, cut into small florets
½ cup rinsed quinoa
½ cup avocado, diced
6 cherry tomatoes
⅓ cucumber, diced
2 green onions
1 cup beans (says Naomi: Two kinds mixed is nice; I
    used kidney and cannellini)
¼ cup loosely packed cilantro or basil
1 teaspoon sesame oil
2 tablespoons rice wine vinegar
juice of half a lime
Pinch sugar, salt, pepper (to taste)

1. Over boiling water, lightly steam the broccoli florets until bright green but still tender, then cool in the refrigerator.

2. In small saucepan with a tight-fitting lid, bring 1 cup of water to a boil. After rinsing the quinoa well, add it to boiling water with a pinch of salt. Turn heat to low and cover. Cook 15 minutes until the water is absorbed. Remove from heat, allow to stand 5 minutes, and fluff with a fork. Place cooked quinoa in a large bowl and set in the fridge to cool.

3. Meanwhile, prep the vegetables and herbs, chopping and cutting as needed.

4. To assemble, add the vegetables to the quinoa and toss gently with the sesame oil, rice wine vinegar, lime juice, and a pinch each of sugar, salt, and pepper.

NOTE: This salad will last a few days in the fridge, but if you are storing it to eat later, don't add the avocado until just before serving.

Adapted from Naomi Pomeroy.

Alex Guarnaschelli's Pea Salad with Basil and Pea Shoots

While she sometimes craves pure, unadorned salads, Alex recognizes that most people like some dressing. The vinaigrette, with three sources of acid and an adjustable amount of oil, would be good on almost any green salad you like. I've dialed down the mustard from Guarnaschelli's recipe; you may add more to taste. Peas are a vegetable that even some green-averse children like—the tiny amount of sugar and the pea shoots make the pea flavor even more pronounced—and the milder dressing should appeal.

serves 4 to 6 as a side dish

2 teaspoons Dijon mustard

1 tablespoon fresh lemon juice

1 tablespoon sherry vinegar

1 tablespoon capers

2 teaspoons caper brine

Salt and freshly ground pepper

⅓ cup extra-virgin olive oil

¼ cup chopped fresh tarragon, washed, dried, and stems removed

Granulated sugar, as needed (she recommends superfine, which dissolves quickly)

8 ounces snow peas, washed, ends trimmed

¾ cup shelled spring (English) peas

8 ounces sugar snap peas, washed, ends trimmed

¼ cup basil leaves, stemmed, washed, dried

¼ cup pea shoots, washed and dried

1. In a medium bowl, whisk together the Dijon mustard, lemon juice, and sherry vinegar. Add the capers, caper brine, and a pinch of salt and pepper to taste. Slowly whisk in the olive oil and add the tarragon. Taste and season with salt and pepper, if needed. Set aside.

2. Bring a large pot of water to a boil over medium heat. Add salt until the water tastes like seawater; then add a generous pinch of sugar.

3. Prepare an ice bath. Fill a large bowl halfway with ice cubes and add some cold water. Put a colander squarely inside the ice bath. The colander will keep you from having to pick the peas out from among the ice cubes in the ice bath.

4. Cook the peas: Add the snow peas to the boiling water and cook until they are bright green and tender, about 1 to 2 minutes. Remove the peas from the water with a strainer and transfer them to the ice bath. Allow them to sit until cooled. Drain on a kitchen towel–lined plate.

5. Bring the water back up to a boil and add the shelled peas. Cook until the water comes back to a boil, about 1 minute. Use the strainer to remove the peas and plunge them into the ice bath. Allow them to sit until cooled. Discard the blanching water.

6. Remove the peas from the ice bath and spread them out onto the kitchen towel over a flat surface. Use another kitchen towel to gently pat them dry. Transfer the towel to a plate and put the peas into the refrigerator to chill until you are ready to serve.

7. Transfer the chilled shelled peas, snow peas, and raw sugar snap peas to a medium bowl. Stir to blend. Toss with the vinaigrette, basil leaves, and pea shoots and season with salt, to taste. Transfer the salad to a platter and serve immediately.

Adapted from Alex Guarnaschelli.

Ming Tsai's Pork Fried Rice

serves 4

Canola oil for cooking
2 garlic cloves, finely chopped
1 tablespoon finely chopped fresh ginger
1 onion, cut into small dice
3 carrots, grated, or 1 cup of carrot nubs, sliced
1 bunch scallions, thinly sliced, white and green
  separated
1 pound ground pork
5 cups cold cooked brown-and-white-rice combo,
  preferably day-old so it's nice and dry (alter-
  natively, place cooked rice on a sheet tray and
  place in freezer to cool and dry)
1 tablespoon of naturally brewed soy sauce
Kosher salt and freshly ground black pepper

1. In a wok or nonstick sauté pan over high heat, add a touch of oil, garlic, and ginger, and stir-fry until soft, about 30 seconds.

2. Add onions, carrot, and scallion whites and stir-fry 3 minutes until al dente—cooked through but not too soft.

3. Add the ground pork and cook until pork colors and is thoroughly cooked (about 8 minutes).

4. Add rice; stir-fry until heated through. Season with soy sauce, kosher salt, and freshly ground black pepper and taste to adjust seasonings.

5. Transfer to a platter, garnish with green scallions, and serve immediately.

Adapted from Ming Tsai.

BEHIND THE LESSONS:

Michael Psilakis's Emotion on a Plate

Michael Psilakis's mother wept openly when he told her that he was skipping law school to become a chef. "I told her, 'I'm going to own a restaurant!' She cried and said, 'That's what your grandfather did!' That's not the way it's supposed to go. Anybody who comes from an immigrant family, they want progress."

Psilakis's father was a fur trader. "When the Greeks came over here they either went into the food industry or the fur industry. I worked with him for many years as a child, and unfortunately the fur industry fell apart in this country, probably when I was about fifteen. That was a trying experience for us. We lost a lot. It was a struggle."

So his degree in accounting and plan to go to law school was seen as a triumph. But for Psilakis, "Becoming a chef was sort of natural, because food was always something that was not only very enjoyable to me, but also something that I really loved to be able to give to people. For most chefs, food is a gift and allows us to create what we feel inside emotionally, and transfer that to a plate and give it to someone." Once it was clear to his parents that he was on his way to being a star chef, not a struggling restaurant cook, "they were happy."

When his father died in 2007, he says, "I realized how much he and I communicated with food. I started writing to deal with his passing, writing down all these stories about moments we spent together, and I realized food kept coming up as a common theme in these stories. I decided to write a cookbook as an homage to him and my family." Food is one way many people connect to their loved ones. But for Psilakis, it goes further. "Fine dining for me is also a means of expressing an emotional connection; I just use food as a medium to communicate that," he tells me. "So you use a pen, and I'm using a piece of meat." It's an interesting proposition: While everyone understands how a comforting family recipe evokes a loved one's memory, a chef has a much higher bar, trying to emotionally reach hordes of anonymous diners who pull up to his restaurant tables each night.

Psilakis had the opportunity to reach out on an unusually grand scale in 2009, when he was invited to cook at the White House for Greek Independence Day. "The only thing I can liken it to was if you got a medal in the Olympics and you stood on a podium and heard your national anthem." It was an outsize expression of the sort of progress for which his immigrant parents had hoped. While his father wasn't there to see it, he did get many letters from Greek-Americans, strangers to him, voicing their joy. While he thinks often about how what he puts on a plate affects a diner, he hadn't anticipated his own emotional response. "It blindsided me: I had a sense of pride that I didn't really expect."

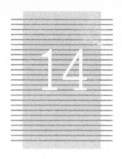

EAT AS IF YOUR LIFE DEPENDS ON IT

COOKING IS TRANSFORMATION. Bring together ingredients: wet, dry, yeasty, milky, eggy, and somehow—through science, although seemingly through magic—they become something else: bread or cake or a popover.

Food also transforms the body, practically on contact. It can make you feel energized or sluggish. Over time, it can build strength through sustenance, or it can wreak havoc. I think I've always wanted food to do too much. I want it to nourish me and help keep me healthy, to give me energy and not weigh me down. I want it to satisfy me both physically and emotionally. I want it to create bonds and shared memories within my family; no one ever got misty-eyed remembering his mother's salad dressed only with lemon juice. There has to be a place for both spare, healthy meals and for all-out comfort eating.

And I will always believe that cooking can be transformed from a mundane daily chore into an expression of love. But I worry when that love goes awry, when a passion for food turns into overeating—or worse, when it contributes to poor health. That, by their own admissions, was the case for some chefs I spoke with. Too much food, or too much of the wrong food, or just too much muchness.

No one would have guessed from looking at him that Simpson Wong, a slender Malaysian-born chef in New York, was a heart-attack candidate—and that includes him. Then just forty-two years old, he had been to the gym and to work at his South Asian restaurant; he ended the day in the hospital having an angioplasty. Once he came to terms with that reality, he knew what had been the likely cause: a family history, paired with stress (he had just opened a second restaurant), smoking, and eating a lot of fat- and cholesterol-laden foods, which described a lot of his old favorites.

Wong and the other chefs in this chapter share what I think are remarkable stories of starting over. "Being overweight is one thing," says Alex Stratta, who lost over a hundred pounds after a cancer diagnosis. "But looking at possibly not making it through the year is something else." Michael Psilakis didn't have the shock of a major health crisis, but his body ached under the extra weight it was carrying, and he knew he could not continue down the path he was on. If working around food and staying slim is challenging, it is nothing compared to working around food and actively losing a lot of weight. Not all of the methods described here will speak to everybody, but each chef offers a frank look at how he remade his body and his life.

Lesson 85: **Michael Psilakis's Un–Middle Way**

"Food is used on so many different levels: to help relieve stress, or as a prize for a job well-done, or just self-gratification that is immediate and easy," says Psilakis. The first time I met him, I wouldn't have suspected he ever had a weight problem. But he proved it: He pulled out his old driver's license. It was, I imagine, like carrying a Dorian Gray portrait around with you at all times—an alternate Psilakis, the one before he made over not just his appearance, but his entire relationship to food.

"In the household that I grew up in, food was central to everything we did. So eating brings you back to fond memories. It becomes an addiction for a lot of people. I definitely fall into that category." Simply put, he says, "I blew up."

At his top weight, when he was in his mid-thirties, Psilakis was over three hundred pounds. He describes the way he ate as having no boundaries. "Being a chef is a difficult profession in the sense that you work all day to cook this really beautiful food for people, but you yourself very rarely sit down to eat. So you find yourself picking all day—it's part of your job." He did his job well: Although the well-regarded Anthos closed, he soon launched three more restaurants. "Opening a restaurant, I easily gain twenty pounds. Easily, just from recipe testing. No exaggeration, I'll eat ten thousand calories a day."

At home he was also eating big. "My family had that philosophy of, 'You have to clean your plate,' something you find in most immigrant families—you can't waste any of this. The reality is that we should eat only what we need to make ourselves happy, and then stop. But with me, if I enjoyed the way something tasted, I would just eat until I was sick. Or it would be twelve o'clock at night and I would be taking hamburgers out of the freezer and going outside and grilling—and not because I was hungry. No, I just had dinner two hours before. But I'm highly suggestible." He would see the frozen burgers and suddenly a midnight cookout for one seemed like a good idea. "That's the thing that people have to be realistic about: Are they really hungry when they're eating these things?"

Besides the poor eating, "I was doing no exercise, and I was smoking." Standing for up to seventeen hours a day, six or seven days a week, made his knees, feet, and back ache; his only relief came for the few hours he lay down at night. "Your body is not meant to carry that amount of weight all day long. At a certain point you realize that this is not good for you and you have to do something. One day I just said, 'This has to stop.'"

He didn't give up on the profession, obviously. He knew he would have to find a way to change his approach to food, without walking away from the work he so loved. An idea came to him: He would stop eating for three days. Not to lose weight—any weight you lose by fasting you'll put right back on—but as a kind of reset button, a seventy-two-hour line that would divide his old life from his new one. "I fasted for three days. Just water. This is maybe not for everyone. I'm not a doctor; I'm not advocating not eating for three days."

This is a point worth repeating. Do not go on a twenty-four- or forty-eight- or seventy-two-hour or any length fast without talking to a doctor first. It is likely that your doctor will talk you out of it. This is Michael's story, and it is one of extremes, both in the behavior that got him in trouble, and in his initial response to it. When the notion to fast came to him, he knew he could probably do it, because he has each year severely restricted his diet for forty days as part of the Greek Orthodox observance of Lent. "Our tradition was that you wouldn't eat anything that came from an animal that had blood. So there is no meat, no eggs—no dairy at all. You could eat shellfish, and there were a lot of salads and beans and vegetarian things that we ate. Then the last week of Lent it was stricter. You were basically committing yourself to bread and water. We did that every year. So for me to say I'm going to fast for three days is not that outlandish. I wanted to start fresh."

Whether you are compelled or put off by his notion of going without food for three days (and try to imagine doing it while cooking in a restaurant kitchen all the while), it did, somehow, reboot his system, and he began eating as a different man.

Once he made up his mind to change, the physical act of eating less and eating better was, he says, surprisingly easy. "You really have to get yourself in a situation where you're ready to say, 'I'm going to change the way that I use food.' The first hurdle is making the mental commitment."

After that came the external changes. He began eating salads every day, and that is still what he has for lunch almost daily. "A simple salad with different types of proteins. Today I had a salad with chickpeas, tomatoes, black-eyed peas, grilled chicken, roasted peppers, lettuce, and olives."

He decided to drink more water, several glasses throughout the day, and rarely drank anything sweetened, like soda, explaining, "I'd rather eat."

He curbed his late-night eating: After work now, "I'll have a sandwich or my wife will have made some sort of dinner or there's leftover Chinese food. The difference is now I'm taking two spoonsful, not finishing the whole thing."

Mainly he was eating the kind of fresh Greek food he serves: salads, grilled fish, vegetables, house-made yogurts. "I'm lucky in that the food is very healthy. We have the ability to eat a lot of wonderful things without throwing butter on it or heavy cream. Those ingredients are not really in our kitchen."

One thing Psilakis refused to do was to make a forbidden-foods list. He limited bread, his biggest love, but didn't cut it out entirely. This man who used to knock off a Halloween-size bag of M&M's can now eat a small handful and leave it at that. Even pizza he now eats in controlled portions. "Before, I could easily eat eight slices or more. Going to two slices was significant."

His new commitment paid off: He lost more than eighty pounds in six months, which completely reshaped his body. "I lost a shoe size," he marvels. "I mean, think about how big you have to be in order for your foot to shrink—it's not a very fatty part of a body." He also quit smoking. You don't need a doctor's advice to know that's a good idea. Stop.

In the midst of all this transformation, however, where were the workouts that so many other big-losing chefs find essential? "You notice I never mentioned exercise, really," says Psilakis. "That's my biggest flaw: Every once in a while I start, but it's time-consuming, and not something I really enjoy, which is a problem. I have to physically will my way through it. As I'm getting older, it seems more necessary, because just maintaining portion size doesn't bring you back."

He has found joy in being active with his son. "I hadn't participated in any sports since I was a kid until my son forced me to. Now I'm back into it, playing soccer with him over the weekend." His new size makes that kind of bonding possible. But kicking around a ball with a youngster doesn't always qualify as a sweaty workout.

Maybe the secret is this: As much as he dislikes exercise, Psilakis craves competition. When some of his younger staff members decided to train for a triathlon, he got in on the action. "I love when somebody puts a challenge in front of me." He did it—he completed the race. How? I asked. How did you go from nonathlete to triathlete? The practical answer is that he trained hard every day for sixty to ninety minutes, for six months. The deeper answer, and one that better explains how Psilakis achieved his weight loss: "I'm very goal driven. The middle road, to me, has always been somewhat boring, I guess."

Lesson 86: Simpson Wong knows it isn't only calories that count

It seemed as if Simpson Wong, the chef at Café Asean and Wong, could eat anything. He was naturally slender, and whatever nature didn't burn off, he did with a combination of workouts, cigarettes, and stress. Without having to think about calories, he indulged frequently in favorite foods: late-night burgers and fries, and in the morning, big bowls of pork ramen or of laksa, a cholesterol-heavy coconut curry soup with noodles, egg, and a deep-fried tofu puff. That, he notes, was consumed after "a whole night of tasting sauce, with salt and fat and bone marrow and red wine reduced until it is concentrated. It adds up."

In January 2003 he had opened a new restaurant, Jefferson, that quickly became a Greenwich Village place to be seen. (Television trivialists will remember it as the location of Miranda and Steve's wedding reception on *Sex and the City*.) Five months later, on Friday, May 13, Wong felt a tightness in his chest after using the weight machines at his gym. "The way I had been eating and drinking, I thought it was acid reflux," he says. He walked to the pharmacy, bought an antacid, and had just enough time to pop one in his mouth before he dropped to the floor. Another customer offered to call an ambulance, but Wong got up and continued his day, walking toward the farmers' market. Some celebrity guests—a network head and his famous wife—were to be at Jefferson that night, and he wanted to prepare a special dinner.

"In half a block, the pain was back. So I took myself to the restaurant and my manager gave me some Pepto-Bismol. After I took that I ate a clear soup of egg whites, asparagus, and chicken stock. Still it didn't go away. Then the pain was shooting down my arm. I thought, 'You know, I should go get a massage.'"

Is this the right time to tell you that Wong's longtime boyfriend is a cardiologist?

Eventually the pain became too much and he did call his boyfriend, who told him to get to the hospital. He did, and that night underwent a lifesaving angioplasty.

When he came home, he knew a lot would have to change. He quit smoking, of course, and found that for the first time in his life he was craving a lot of sweets. "After the heart attack I put on weight; I went up to a hundred and fifty-eight. For my size (five-seven) I was very round." He wasn't so concerned with losing the weight, which he did soon after—despite that very bad day at the gym, he remains an exercise fan—but instead with eating a diet that would support his heart health.

"For every meal, I look for omega-3 fatty acid in it; I look for vegetables, for fiber." (Omega-3 fats are healthful unsaturated fats found in walnuts, canola oil, and some types of fish, such as salmon and herring.) "I trim off all the skin, and no fried stuff. I don't remember the last time I had a burger or fried chicken," says Wong. "In restaurants, I try to avoid dishes with hidden fats, like stews. I eat more good stuff: fish, chicken, vegetables. I don't have butter when I go out to dinner. If they bring a basket of bread and some butter, I ask for olive oil. That's a great substitute.

"For a while I was going to vegan places, and I have more interest in Mediterranean and Middle Eastern food now. But I am still a fan of braised pork dishes—you go to Thailand or Malaysia and they use all different parts of the pig: ears, intestines, anything in a stew with sweet soy sauce—now I'll only eat the lean part of it. No coconut milk—some dieticians claim it's actually not that bad for you, but it still has cholesterol in it, and I'm very concerned with cholesterol."

He became newly critical of how restaurants treat their customers' health, though as a chef-owner himself, he knows how profitable the tastiest, fattiest menu items often are. "Isn't it bad," he asks me, over lunch of smoked trout salad (his) and roast chicken salad (mine), "how everywhere you go they have to have a burger on the menu? As long as you have a burger you will get people in." Visiting a friend's restaurant a while ago, he was sent a house special, he recalls, "a foie gras beignet with maple syrup and bacon ice cream. We were at the counter where he was cooking, so naturally you have to eat some of that. He didn't know my history."

Wong was unwilling to pander on his menu. He briefly closed Jefferson to retool its concept, before reopening it as Jefferson Grill, which had lighter fare. "If I was going to be cooking there, I needed to change the menu. I had to come out with something a little bit healthier. No more butter, just a little bit of cream in one dish." Eventually, though, that iteration also closed. He tried to make some tweaks to what he served at Café Asean, but found that "people get mad if I take something off the menu." So the coconut curries are still being served, and the neighborhood spot continues to thrive.

At his newest restaurant, Wong, he serves food he likes to eat, what he calls Asian locavore: "The food I grew up eating in Malaysia, but using local ingredients, and grass-fed beef." Besides being better for you and for the planet, well-aged grass-fed beef is richer and needs little in the way of heavy sauces, which can add lots of fat and calories. He's attracting new customers with innovative dishes—scallops with crispy duck tongue and jellyfish appeared on a debut menu—not with burgers. The food, says Wong, is "as whole and wholesome as possible."

Lesson 87: Alessandro Stratta learned to listen to his body

Alex Stratta is a fifth-generation hotelman; until the age of fourteen he lived in hotels, and says, "I never had the luxury of saying I was from anywhere." He grew up on room service and restaurant meals and started working at age sixteen. "I was always kind of chubby, but I worked out a lot." Once he began opening his own restaurants, he no longer exercised much, but "kept eating like I did," he says. He was running two luxury hotel restaurants, called Alex and Stratta, working hard and living life, and, he says, "The next thing you know, you're 280 pounds."

In 2007, when his then-wife was very pregnant with their twins, Stratta saw his doctor for a scheduled checkup. There, he found out he had colon cancer. "That was the wake-up call that I wasn't taking care of my body. There is no cancer in my family. I believe I brought it on myself—I was eating and drinking whatever I wanted, and copious amounts of both," says Stratta.

Fortunately the cancer was discovered early. Two weeks later his children were born, a boy and a girl. Stratta was treated successfully, but he didn't heed his body's warning immediately; that came only after six months of, as he puts it, "self-pity and shock." Then one of his restaurants was nominated for an award, and Stratta needed a tuxedo for the occasion. At the store, he recalls, "They didn't have anything in my size. That was my 'oh, shit' moment. Your body will tell you to change—whether it's with cancer or with a size-twenty neck."

Soon after, he stopped drinking alcohol and eating much sugar or red meat. "I'd rather have one slice, once in a while, of really rich beef, where you taste the fattiness of the meat, than a lot of lean meat." He cut back on white flours, pastas, most starches, in fact. "I don't care what kind of bread—you can have your sprouted grain or whatever. For me, starch is starch, and I knew it was bad for me because it didn't feel good. If you eat something and fifteen minutes later you don't feel good, that's a sign you shouldn't have put it in your body. After you go from total excess to total discipline and then you cheat, your body tells you."

He returned to workouts, riding his bicycle for an hour a day, five days a week. After his divorce, he began dating a woman who is also a nutritionist and chef. She put him on her program, which included a directive to stop eating for the day by six p.m. "I eat my last meal before dinner service." He gets his tasting done before that, and has become more judicious about how much he tastes. "I dip a spoon. You don't have to taste a whole scallop."

What he did eat was food he loved: fresh seafood, vegetables, and fruit, and occasional sweets in moderation. "If you completely abstain, you will crack. Go a few days, not six months, without ice cream."

Routine became very important to Stratta; it was easier to find a handful of foods that he liked and that fit his new goals than to make choices each day. Breakfast is a fruit-and-protein smoothie. Lunch virtually every weekday is pho from a local Vietnamese place: glass noodles, chicken, and vegetables in broth. Dinner always begins with a big salad of lettuces, celery, tomatoes, and cucumbers dressed in vinegar and olive oil. Then he'll have roasted fish or chicken and some fruit if he's still hungry. He admits, "I do miss the starches a lot. I'm from a Northern Italian family, so it was pasta, it was gnocchi, it was risotto, it was butter, it was cream. Butter, I love. A baguette with butter and prosciutto is . . . *ahhh*. But I can't remember the last time I had that."

With his weight under control, "I feel great. I'm really active with my kids—in the pool in their gym class—it's fantastic; I love it," Stratta tells me as he is heading off to a kiddie gym class with his children. "My son is three and a half going on four; my daughter is three and a half going on fifteen."

Diners at Stratta also got the benefit of his transformation. "I started cooking smarter, healthier. Cream, I haven't used it in my cooking in a long time." His best advice? Don't just *say* you're going to reinvent the way you eat. "It's one thing to say you're not going to eat sugar, flour, fatty meats. It's another to do it. You have to do it."

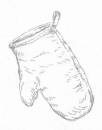

Michael Psilakis's Cretan-spiced Tuna with Bulgur

This is a recipe that you should look at as adaptable separates: The spice blend is good on other fish or chicken, the bulgur salad is good on its own, the vinaigrette could be used on another salad, and the fish could certainly be served with a different side. Note: Bulgur wheat comes in various sizes; prepare it according to package.

serves 4

1 tablespoon extra-virgin olive oil, plus more for
   drizzling
¼ cup minced Spanish or sweet onion
2 cloves garlic, crushed and chopped
1 cup coarse (number 3) bulgur
3 cups water
Kosher salt and cracked black pepper
8 large sun-dried tomatoes, slivered
1 cup golden raisins
1 cup pine nuts
¼ cup capers
24 oil-cured black olives, pitted and chopped
½ cup Greek yogurt
¼ cup distilled white vinegar
Large pinch sweet paprika
2 tablespoons blended oil (Michael uses mostly
   canola with a bit of olive oil added in)
1½ pounds ahi tuna loin, cut into 4 steaks
Cretan spice mix (recipe follows)

Red wine–black pepper vinaigrette (recipe follows)

¼ cup roughly chopped fresh herbs, such as parsley and/or dill

Fresh lemon juice

Sea salt

FOR THE SPICE MIX:

1 teaspoon cumin seeds

1 teaspoon mustard seeds (not black)

1 teaspoon fennel seeds

3 brown cardamom pods, crushed

10 whole black peppercorns

1. Preheat an oven or toaster oven to 350°F. Combine the cumin, mustard, and fennel seeds, the cardamom pods, and the peppercorns on a baking sheet or shallow tray of a toaster oven. Bake for 5 to 10 minutes, until fragrant.

2. Let cool completely; then transfer to a designated spice grinder and process to a fine powder. Store in an airtight container away from light and heat for up to 2 months.

RED WINE–BLACK PEPPER VINAIGRETTE

makes 1¼ cups

½ cup red wine vinegar

1 small grilled onion

6 leaves basil

1 teaspoon picked thyme

2 tablespoons Dijon mustard

6 small cloves garlic, smashed

2 shallots, thickly sliced

2 tablespoons dry Greek oregano

1 tablespoon kosher salt

1 tablespoon coarsely cracked black pepper

¾ cup extra-virgin olive oil

1. In a food processor, combine the vinegar, grilled onion, basil, thyme, mustard, garlic, shallots, oregano, salt, and pepper.

2. With the motor running, drizzle in the olive oil until smooth. Add salt and pepper to taste.

★ To make white wine vinaigrette, substitute white wine vinegar.

TO MAKE THE DISH:

1. In a saucepan, warm the olive oil over medium-low heat. Add the onion and garlic and sauté gently until tender. Add the bulgur and stir over the heat for 2 minutes, to toast slightly.

2. Add the water and a generous amount of kosher salt and pepper. Bring to a boil and remove from the heat. Cover and let stand for 1 hour. Combine the cooked bulgur, sun-dried tomatoes, raisins, pine nuts, capers, and olives. Keep at room temperature.

3. Whisk together the yogurt, vinegar, and paprika. Season with salt and pepper.

4. In a large skillet, warm the blended oil over medium-high heat. Season the tuna on both sides with salt and pepper. Dust all sides generously with the Cretan spice mix. Sear the tuna for about 2 minutes, then turn over, reduce the heat, and cook for 1½ to 2 minutes more, depending on how rare or well-done you like it.

5. Add just enough vinaigrette to dress the bulgur salad lightly. Season with salt and pepper, sprinkle with fresh herbs, and toss.

6. Smear a large spoonful of the yogurt mixture on each of 4 dinner plates. Top with bulgur salad. Cut the tuna into thick slices and place on top of the salad. Drizzle with lemon juice and olive oil. Finish with salt and pepper.

Adapted from *How to Roast a Lamb: New Greek Classic Cooking* by Michael Psilakis. Little, Brown and Company, 2009.

⁓

Alex Stratta's Kombu and Chickpea Soup with Tuscan Kale

This recipe is based on a soup that Stratta used to make at his restaurant, and would often eat for dinner himself. His is a beautifully elevated approach to the Italian peasant-food combo of beans and greens. Adapted with his permission, this version of the dish goes back to its rustic roots, but keeps Stratta's clever addition of Japanese kombu seaweed and togarashi pepper (a widely sold Japanese dried red pepper blend). I assure you, you will use both the kombu (for dashi) and the Japanese pepper (for anything that takes pepper) again.

serves 4

2 cups dried chickpeas
1 piece dried kombu, about 1x4 inches
8 cups vegetable broth

2 cups Tuscan kale (also called lacinato kale),
    washed, tough stems removed, and leaves cut
    into 1-inch pieces
Salt and freshly ground pepper to taste
Togarashi pepper to taste

1. Pick through the chickpeas to remove any stones or debris. Soak 8 hours or overnight in a large bowl, generously covered with cool water.

2. Wipe the kombu with a damp cloth to remove all the excess dried salt and any white film on the seaweed. Place the chickpeas, kombu, and the vegetable stock in a large stockpot and bring to a boil. Reduce the heat to low to maintain a simmer. Cook until chickpeas are tender, about 40 minutes to 1 hour. (Cooking times depend on the age of the beans. Start tasting for doneness at 30 minutes.)

3. Once the chickpeas are cooked, remove from heat and remove the kombu. Strain the chickpeas through a colander set over a large bowl. Reserve the broth.

4. In a blender or food processor, blend half the chickpeas with some of the broth until smooth (you may need to work in batches).

5. Place the chickpeas, whole and blended, as well as enough broth to desired consistency in a saucepan large enough to hold everything. Warm over medium heat and add the kale. Cook until softened, about 10 minutes. Season to taste with salt, pepper, and togarashi pepper.

Adapted from Alex Stratta.

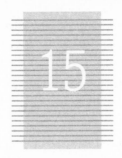

Eat with and Cook for Friends

66 **W**HEN WE FIRST opened Lantern, I had that feeling of, 'Every plate of food represents you.' I remember going into the dining room when someone didn't like their chicken and asking, 'What didn't you like?'" recalls Andrea Reusing. "You want to please every person. When is the food exactly the way you want it? Never. You can always make it better, and finding the line is hard."

This, essentially, is how I feel about hosting dinner parties. Of course, at home you don't have the option of hiding in the kitchen; you have to sit down and eat with your guests. Despite their camaraderie, dinner parties are the closest most of us non-chefs will come to knowing what it is to cook for customers. That can be a lot of pressure. Particularly if you're blessed to live in a city with more restaurants than a person could fully experi-ence in a lifetime, can a compelling argument even be made for spending a free evening eating other people's home cooking? Is there any culinary reason friends should come to your house?

Beyond the stress of contemplating those questions, cooking for friends is a subversive idea when you're trying to keep your eating in check. Everyone knows you eat more when you're around the table talking, laughing, and topping off one another's wine glasses. And since you want guests to say, "This is delicious," not, "This is pretty good for a low-fat dish," there's always the temptation to bring out the butter and go crazy—their diets are not your problem, right?

Plenty of chefs had suggestions for cooking for others at home without falling into that trap. Master a couple of them, and your take on dinner parties might change. "There is this natural joy and instant gratification that you get from making something with your hands and putting it together for somebody," says Sue Torres. "It's a very intimate and personal thing."

Entertaining doesn't have to upset your own healthy regimen—in fact, it can improve it. "I eat a lot better when I'm cooking for someone else," says Rick Moonen. "If I'm alone, I have ramen once a week, because I'm not inspired to cook for myself." By inviting company over, he says, "I keep protein in the house, not just ramen." If you've been going through a cereal-for-dinner phase, or a Chinese takeout rut, inviting a few friends over for a real meal can break a bad-eating streak.

Lesson 88: Smart chefs cook the way they like to eat

"I love to have people over," says Gregory Gourdet. But he is the first to say he doesn't eat like a typical chef. When he goes out with friends, he admits, "It is kind of annoying to be with

me, actually. In the chef world you're supposed to eat everything, and I am sort of picky." Not to worry. If you've taken up
eating more healthfully, there's no reason not to share your new
enthusiasm with your friends. Assuming that you're cooking
and eating real food, it is bound to be good.

Since cutting most dairy, red meat, and refined carbohydrates
from his diet, Gourdet has figured out how to prepare meals
that don't leave him or most guests missing those elements. "I
feel empowered when I know I am making something as delicious and as healthy as possible. I feel like I am doing something
amazing for my body and for my friends' health when I cook
for them as well." The night before we spoke, Gourdet had just
had some people over. On the menu: roast chicken (See? What
did I tell you about roast chicken?) with chili flakes, lemon, and
rosemary from his garden; a frittata; and roasted vegetables:
sweet potatoes, onions, whole garlic cloves, and parsnips cooked
with lots of chilies. Roasting vegetables until they are well caramelized is another way to boost flavor without much fat (just
a drizzling of oil). Because Gourdet isn't dogmatic about dessert, he served four different cakes from a bakery. Laughing, he
tells me, "It's good to keep a balance."

At home, Marcus Samuelsson says, he has "a badass grill and
a badass kitchen." Professionally, he has cooked Scandinavian,
Japanese, and regional American. His own home-cooking
memories are of Swedish food, though he has also spent time
exploring the cuisine of Ethiopia, where his roots are. So what
does he most often prepare for guests? "Ethiopian food, because
so many people haven't had that outside of a restaurant setting,"
he tells me. "But it is not the same in someone's house." He and
his wife are often in the kitchen together, and for company,
"We might do chicken stew, beef tartare, cottage cheese—you
take buttermilk and bring it to a boil and let it break, strain it,

add toasted mustard leaves for flavor, very simple. Then we'll mix it up with gravlax and meatballs. There's no other house in the world on that day that you can have that meal."

I was greatly inspired by this story in two ways: first to make that chicken stew, called doro we't. (The recipe follows.) Second, I think Marcus makes a good point: Everyone should cook the specialties of his house, whatever they are, even if they don't typically appear together on a menu.

Lesson 89: They take guests' dietary concerns into consideration

Marc Murphy loves cooking for guests at his family's beach house; for much of the season all the guest bedrooms are filled. When he's planning dinners there, his first consideration is usually his wife, Pamela. "I have a wife who doesn't like me cooking much with butter. She doesn't like butter. And I have what I call my 'second wife,' her best friend, and they're both always there. She claims to not like butter either."

I don't know anyone who doesn't like butter. But Marc knows two people; what are the odds? Nonetheless, he is thoughtful about cooking when Pamela and her friend are his target audience. He'll prepare some of his favorites, but adapt them. For instance, at his restaurant Landmarc, he might serve a pork-chop dish with caramelized apples and onions, sautéed spinach, and a bordelaise sauce (red wine, butter, etc.). "At the beach, I'll do that same dish with the apples, onions, and spinach, but I do a sauce of herbs, olive oil, and splash of vinegar on the pork."

When in doubt, go lighter: Use vegetable stock if you have vegetarians among your crowd. Don't offer up obvious diet-busters, or so few options that people might find themselves in a bind over eating what you're serving. Even if you know your audience, it's great to give options. Nancy Silverton often entertains a friendly pack of carnivores around her backyard grill. "I'll do hamburgers, steaks, sausages, or lamb chops, anything really easy. I always like to accompany any of those with condiments that are wonderful spooned on: a romesco or a pesto or a tapenade. I always serve colorful bowls of condiments. I can sort of personalize the food. It adds flavor. I enjoy eating that way," she says. That's important too: Serve food you love.

Lesson 90: They think about the rhythm of a meal

As much as you want to get that "yum" from your friends, cooking for guests doesn't have to be an orgy of slick, buttery, love-me foods. "Don't choose all showstoppers," says Rick Bayless, who cooked for the nation's ultimate dinner party, a White House state dinner, when the guest of honor was Mexican president Felipe Calderón.

"Start with simpler flavors; then go to the boldest stuff at the end," he advises. And think about texture: "You don't want to have two things in a row with a creamy texture—pair something creamy with something that has a crunch. I want the first flavors to be bright, with pizzazz to them, something exciting. At the White House we started out with a very simple dish: a jicama-and-orange salad—no meat or fish on it. Light, bright flavors, crunch, cilantro on there, a little bit of red chili that whets your appetite. Then we went to a ceviche dish, again bright, but that had some roasted garlic and roasted green chili, so that gave it a more savory, rounded quality. The main course was a beef dish with a grand mole from Oaxaca. Then dessert, a rich but small tart of Mexican chocolate and goat-milk cara-mel called cajeta. It wasn't overwhelming."

Translated: a little crispy salad, a virtually uncooked fish dish (a recipe for ceviche by Laurent Gras follows), a one-pot dish of which you're proud, and a little dessert. Done—a meal good enough to serve at the White House, or your own.

Lesson 91: They cook casually off duty

Sang Yoon, who wants nothing more than to cook for you at his restaurants, loathes entertaining at home. "I rarely have people over. Maybe once a year. I'm not a party guy," says Yoon. "And I hate the holidays. I usually hide during the holidays. I used to have something called 'Sangsgiving,' because I hate turkey. If I have a day off, I don't want to eat dry poultry. It's a punishment. Is this my day of atonement? I used to take matters into my own hands and make a big rib roast or roast a whole lobe of foie gras—now, this is a celebration! I did that a few years, but it became too much work, so now I go out for Chinese food."

But I found that Yoon is singular among chefs in this regard—most love to cook for their friends and family. Among the most impassioned is Michael Psilakis, who routinely has an informal collection of ten or twelve people over on his days off. "I don't see life being worth living if you don't have that. Why just go home and . . . what, eat? Then sit in front of the TV? Why not say every night you're going to have someone come over and spend time with them? Think about the memories that you have in life—the good ones—and then think about how many of those you could probably associate with what you were eating."

"I love cooking at home," says Sue Torres. "I wish someone would clean up after me, because I can make a mess. But I'm a big fan of using the grill in the summer, spring, fall, for vegetables, meat, chicken, fish. In the winter and the fall, it's more like 'one-pot wonders.' I'll make lentil chili, or beef stew."

Three different chefs (none with Spanish restaurants) mentioned that they like making paella for guests—it's showy without being impossible, and there's only one big pan to clean when you're done. "I made one recently and everyone ate it again for breakfast the next morning," says Cat Cora.

Jacques Torres spends the warmer months living on a boat in a slip on the Hudson River. Without having seen your kitchen, I can guarantee that a boat galley is smaller. With a one-dish meal, he says, "I'm set up on the boat to cook for the whole dock, for twenty people. I have a huge pan to make paella. Every Sunday in the summer my family used to eat outside, a big party. I miss that. If friends are on the dock, I'll make lunch: one brings wine; one brings fruit; one brings a salad." Torres is a casual-dining proponent, but only to a point: "We use those disposable plates. Well, except for me. I don't eat on a disposable dish. I'm not a snob; I just hate how the cardboard flops, and the Styrofoam doesn't sound right. I'm the only person who has glass on a boat—usually you don't, in case you take a big wave. You know what? I'll buy a new glass. I don't want to drink my wine in a plastic container; it's disgusting. My friends laugh at me, but that's the way I like to do it."

Hear, hear!

Lesson 92: Okay, smart chefs employ a few restaurant tricks at home

A pause for a true-life fable.

One of the most peculiar and most enjoyable interviews I've

ever conducted was with the pioneering avant-garde Spanish chef Ferran Adrià, when he was visiting New York on the occasion of the U.S. release of his book *A Day at El Bulli*. I arrived to find another chef joining us, José Andrés, who had been mentored by Adrià, and now is famed in his own right for his five restaurants in Washington, D.C., and the Bazaar in L.A. I hadn't come prepared to interview them both, and was thinking about how to wing this when Andrés greeted me and said that he was here only as a translator for Adrià. This is like showing up to interview Balanchine to find that Baryshnikov is there to interpret. (Yes, I realize Balanchine is dead; work with me.) It was extraordinary. But both chefs were game and friendly, despite the fact that Adrià (whose usual interpreter, Lucy, was on a break) had already endured several journalists, one of whom insisted on taking him to the Lower East Side for pastrami and egg creams. How was he holding up? I asked. "Interviews," he told me, "are a good way to save money, not having to go to the psychotherapist."

Our conversation didn't immediately dig that deep into his psyche—what I was mainly interested in was whether any of the techniques he pioneered at El Bulli could be adapted for regular folk to attempt. How could I impress some dinner party guests without access to a nitrogen tank? Of the more than five hundred pages in his book, did none of them have something practical to say to the home cook? Here, he got politely agitated. After I had asked the question a few ways, Andrés at last told me: "He says: When he buys a book about architecture, he doesn't build a house."

The moral? You are not a restaurant chef. When your friends come over they want to eat well, but they don't expect plates to be Jackson Pollocked with coulis from a squeeze bottle or precious, precarious towers of what Art Smith calls "tepee food." Still, there are a few tricks to borrow from restaurant chefs from their cook–at–home playbooks.

• **Customize your space.** A miniature home kitchen is no excuse for not cooking big. Tom Colicchio is used to working in the roomy and well-laid-out Craft space. But his apartment kitchen is no larger than mine (he can't open his refrigerator all the way, because it hits the oven). And counter space in New York City? *Fugetaboutit.* My own first New York apartment had its "kitchen" in a converted closet, with about two feet of counter space, most of that taken up by a small microwave (a dinner plate wouldn't fit inside) and a single-burner hot plate. Reader, I cooked.

To overcome the space issues, before prepping a big meal, Colicchio says, "I take out things like the toaster, the dish rack. It all goes into the other room." I am embarrassed to admit that it took Colicchio pointing out that I could unplug and move appliances I'm not using. But, voilà, more counter space.

• *Mise en place*—French for having your *merde* together. Essential when cooking with vegetables that need peeling, dicing, and so on. "Organization is it: Once you get to the stove, you're not chopping anymore; that all happens early on," instructs Colicchio. "Get small plastic containers; put your *mise en place* in there; get it all organized."

• **Use all your senses**—and trust them more than whatever cookbook you've got open. Does the food smell done? Does it look done? Does it crunch, crackle, sizzle? Does it spring back or sag when you poke it? Even if you are using a recipe, trust yourself. (The Marx Brothers' rule: "Who you gonna believe: me or your own eyes?") Don't leave something on the stove because a recipe told you to cook it for ten minutes; your nose, eyes, ears, and fingers might tell you different. Finally, taste what you're making. That's what the instruction "season to taste" in a recipe means—you have to taste your food and decide whether it needs more salt, a splash more acid, something herbal, or the bite of peppers. Trust that you aren't going to be "wrong" about this—if it tastes good to you, it tastes good. Need more convincing? If you've ever watched a TV cooking competition, you know people get sent home for putting out food they haven't tasted. Don't have your guests conspiring to vote you off—taste before you serve.

But remember that when you're watching what you eat, you need to watch all those bites in the kitchen too. If you're conscious of it, you might find that you've eaten the equivalent of a small meal during the preparation. "If I'm in my house cooking for people, I'm tasting all the time," says Marc Murphy. "By the time I sit down, I'm ready for my glass of wine, but I'll just watch everybody else. I'll serve myself, but it's hard to sit down and eat."

• **Enjoy the process.** For Christmas Eve, Colicchio has his family over, a dozen or so guests, and prepares a traditional Italian feast of thirteen fishes. "My grandmother used to do it, and I took it over. It's not thirteen dishes, just thirteen fish. I do *fritto misto*, little whitebait and Nantucket bay scallops; sole with lemon, fennel, parsley, capers, red onion sliced really thin; then a *crudo* of tuna with a truffle vinaigrette and lardo; grilled sardines with a sweet-sour onion-and-raisin relish; a raw hamachi with a preserved lemon vinaigrette; salt cod, steamed and flaked, with olive oil, parsley, garlic; a beet salad with anchovies and artichokes and celery, hot cherry peppers, olive oil, parsley, garlic; then we do cacciucco [an Italian fish stew; he uses squid, clams, tomatoes], roast cod with preserved lemon and olives, and pasta."

Phew. If you're planning to cook that much, you had better have a good time doing it, and Colicchio does. "I do it all my-

self. Well, I cheat a little: I have the fish filleted at the restaurant."
(Note: This is not cheating; you do not have to fillet your own
fish.) "I wake up in the morning, get a pot of coffee going, put
music on. I start cooking at ten in the morning and don't stop
until the guests walk in. I don't rush. I enjoy it."

This is welcome advice: Enjoy wonderful food, including the
process of putting it together, especially for loved ones.

I take that sentiment to heart on the afternoon of New Year's
Eve, as I start to assemble dinner for seven. I head to the grocery
store with a plan in my head, and a shopping list based around
a couple of recipes. Though I've never tried it before, I decide
I'm going to roast a duck with lots of root vegetables (carrots,
parsnips—whatever looks good at the store) and apples. Because it is a holiday, this once-in-a-while treat seems in order. I
know it isn't wise to cook a high-bar dish like duck for company when you've never attempted it, but I've roasted a lot of
chickens in the past year, and I'm feeling up to it. Also, I won't
lie: I think it will impress my friends.

I improvise a salad of mixed greens, pear, toasted walnuts, and
mustard-agave vinaigrette. It is meant to be mustard-and-honey
dressing, but alas, I forget to put honey on my list and don't
want to go out again with the duck already blasting away in the
oven. For a side dish I make spaghetti with chopped egg, scallions, butter, and salmon roe, a variation on a long-ago New York
Times recipe that calls for ossetra—an unfunded mandate, if
there ever was one. I won't try to fool you that the fat orange
eggs can pass as the black seed-pearl delight that is real caviar,
although this was not only cheaper, but sustainably raised, so I
felt fine with the substitution. Because no one (until now, I
suppose) knew how the recipe was written, they thought this
was how it was meant to be eaten, with briny, squishy dots
mingling with the chopped hard-boiled egg.

Our neighbors bring sardines grilled with thyme for a first course, and a lemon-coconut cake for dessert. My kid digs into the pungent, oily fish, and encourages his friend to do the same, first telling him, "It's good," and then extolling the sardine's true appeal to a grade-schooler: "Look, it still has an eyeball!"

I hope you don't find it immodest of me to report that the duck comes out phenomenally. Crispy, fatty, skin as brown as a berry, and, as I had hoped, received with great enthusiasm and kudos by my friends as I carry it to the table on a turquoise Fiesta-ware platter that had been waiting for such an occasion. Then I realize I haven't any idea how to carve a duck, never having done it before. The legs are short and the body is long, almost rectangular, with few of the signposts of a chicken or a turkey. Fortunately, another friend has some experience with this, and I hand over the knife, slip into my seat, and become a guest at my own table.

We're fed, happy, some of us giddy with wine, and we talk and laugh over the annual tradition of watching a Marx Brothers movie. At midnight, the kids are still up, and we all gather around the television like it's a hearth to watch the ball drop over Times Square, asking, as we do every year, Who would be crazy enough to stand in that crowd in the cold? The countdown begins and I dash back to the kitchen for a big bowl of red grapes, so that after all the kissing and good wishes we can share in the Spanish custom of eating twelve grapes in the first minute of the New Year. It's a gesture to bring good luck. Reviving and wholesome, it also feels like the best first thing to eat as the calendar turns to a new page and a fresh start.

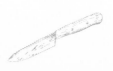

Laurent Gras's Halibut Ceviche with Jalapeño and Parsley

serves 4 as an appetizer

Zest of 1 lime

1 large jalapeño, cut in half lengthwise, stem and
 seeds removed

⅓ cup fresh orange juice

1½ tablespoons fresh lime juice

8 ounces halibut fillet, skin removed, and trimmed
 of any dark spots

Sea salt to taste

2 tablespoons minced flat-leaf (Italian) parsley

Extra-virgin olive oil for serving

1. Chill 4 small bowls in the refrigerator.

2. Zest the lime before juicing it. Set the lime zest aside.

3. Thinly slice one jalapeño half and place in a small bowl with the orange juice and lime juice. Let sit for 30 minutes. In the meantime, dice the remaining jalapeño half to a fine dice. Cut the halibut into ¼-inch pieces and place in a small bowl, set into a larger bowl filled with ice.

4. Strain the jalapeños from the juice through a fine mesh strainer and discard the jalapeño. Lightly season the halibut with sea salt. Add half the citrus juice to the halibut; stir well to combine. Let sit (still resting in bowl of ice) for 5 minutes. Drain the halibut from the citrus juice.

5. Divide the halibut among the chilled bowls. Divide the rest of the citrus juice over each portion of the fish; sprinkle each with the jalapeño, parsley, a little sea salt. Pour a few drops of olive oil and sprinkle a little lime zest over each serving. Serve immediately.

Adapted from Laurent Gras.

Marcus Samuelsson's Doro We't

Two things: First, when I made this I couldn't believe how much chopped onion it called for—it really seemed like a lot. After I had diced up a huge pile (but before I started cooking), I thought, *Next time, I will certainly use less onion.* In fact, the onions cook for more than ninety minutes and melt into a much more reasonable portion of sweet, glazy deliciousness. Second, this recipe calls for berbere, an Ethiopian spice blend that is essential to its character. Jarred is absolutely fine: You can find it at some markets and specialty stores, or online (zamourispices. com). If you don't feel like hunting for it, make your own (Marcus's recipe follows). While berbere has several components, none of them are, individually, hard to find, and you may have some in your drawer already.

Whether you buy or blend, please don't wait until the next time you make this chicken stew to use your berbere again. Its complex mix of peppery heat and sweet notes like cinnamon is great on vegetables or proteins that you are cooking fast on a weeknight. Treat yourself as well as you do your guests! In fact, make extra stew—it freezes well. When I made it for my husband we skipped the cheese and eggs and still had a feast of the aromatic chicken and greens; he liked it even more the next day.

serves 4

¼ cup olive oil

5 garlic cloves, minced

5 small red onions, finely chopped

2-inch piece of ginger, peeled and minced

1 tablespoon tomato paste

3 tablespoons berbere

8 chicken legs, skin removed

1 teaspoon ground cardamom

1 tablespoon salt

3 tablespoons butter

3 cups chicken stock

1 cup dry red wine

1 pound collard greens

4 eggs, hard-boiled and peeled

½ cup cottage cheese (not nonfat)

1. Heat the olive oil in a Dutch oven over low heat. Add the garlic, onions, and ginger and cook, stirring occasionally, until softened, about 30 minutes. Add the tomato paste and berbere and cook for another 15 minutes.

2. Season the chicken legs with the cardamom and salt. Add the chicken to the sauce, along with the butter, stock, and wine. Bring to a simmer and cook until the chicken is cooked through, about 1 hour.

3. In a separate pot, bring salted water to a boil. Add the collard greens and cook until tender, about 15 minutes. Remove the greens with a slotted spoon and transfer to the chicken stew. Serve the stew with hard-boiled eggs and cottage cheese on the side.

Adapted from *New American Table* by Marcus Samuelsson.
John Wiley & Sons, 2009.

BERBERE

1 teaspoon fenugreek seeds
½ cup ground dried chilies
½ cup ground paprika
2 tablespoons salt
2 teaspoons ground ginger
2 teaspoons onion powder
1 teaspoon ground cardamom, preferably freshly
   ground
1 teaspoon ground nutmeg
½ teaspoon garlic powder
¼ teaspoon ground cloves
¼ teaspoon ground cinnamon
¼ teaspoon ground allspice

1. Finely grind the fenugreek seeds with a spice or coffee grinder, or mortar and pestle (you can also start with ground fenugreek and skip this step).

2. Stir together with remaining ingredients in a small bowl. Will keep in a spice jar or tin for months.

Adapted from *Soul of a New Cuisine* by Marcus Samuelsson.
John Wiley & Sons, 2006.

Marc Murphy's Paella

The summer that Murphy bought a paella pan, he used it often for cooking on the grill at the beach. I made this for friends on my apartment stove, using two smaller pans. It made a whole lot, and I was thrilled when our guests readily accepted my offer to take leftovers home and e-mailed me the next day to say they had eaten it for lunch.

serves 6

½ cup extra-virgin olive oil

6 bone-in, skin-on chicken thighs (5 to 6 ounces each)

Salt and freshly ground pepper

1 large white onion, diced

1 red bell pepper or 6 piquillo peppers, seeded and diced

2 garlic cloves, minced

16 ounces (1 pound) short-grain rice, such as Calasparra, bomba, or arborio

1 large pinch saffron

1 cup canned, crushed tomato

5 to 6 cups chicken or seafood broth, plus more as needed

12 littleneck clams, scrubbed

12 mussels, scrubbed

12 medium shrimp, peeled and deveined

1 cup frozen peas

Lemon wedges for serving

1. In a large paella pan or skillet over medium-high heat, warm the olive oil. Season the chicken thighs on both sides with salt and pepper. Cook the chicken skin-side down until browned and crispy, about 5 minutes. Turn over and cook until lightly browned, about 3 to 4 minutes. Remove the chicken to a plate.

2. Reduce the heat to medium and add the onion, peppers, and garlic. Cook until softened and the onions are beginning to turn translucent, about 5 minutes. Add the rice, stir to coat the rice with the oil, and cook until the grains are lightly toasted, about 2 to 3 minutes. Add the saffron and tomato, and cook until the tomatoes have reduced, about 1 minute.

3. Add 5 cups broth. Cook (without stirring) until rice starts to soften, about 10 minutes. Add more broth as needed if the rice is drying out too quickly. Nestle the clams in the rice and, once they begin to open, after about 10 minutes, add the mussels, shrimp, and peas. Cook until the mussels have opened, the shrimp turn pink, and the peas are warmed through, about 5 minutes. Let stand for 15 minutes. Garnish with lemon wedges and serve.

Adapted from Marc Murphy.

Gregory Gourdet's Roasted Vegetables with Olive Oil, Ginger, and Chili

From Gregory: "This is my go-to vegetable dish. I change the vegetables sometimes, based on the season. Squash in the fall, with apples or pears. Maybe asparagus during spring. Use whatever looks good. Stick to dark vegetables and fruits with high nutritional content. Leave the skin on the vegetables. The ginger and chili add some punch and antioxidants."

serves 6

3 large yams, skin on, washed, cut into ¾-inch
    spears (use a mix of garnet yam and jewel yam)
4 slender carrots, tops trimmed, skin on, scrubbed
1 bunch broccolini, bottoms trimmed
2 parsnips, skin on, washed, sliced into wedges
1 medium red onion, peeled, sliced ½-inch thick
1 heads garlic, peeled, whole cloves
1 bunch scallions, trimmed, cut into 1-inch pieces
1 small knob ginger, peeled and minced
1 small red jalapeño, washed, sliced (use whole for
    spicy, half for medium heat)
Sea salt
Olive oil
Cilantro sprigs to garnish

1. Preheat oven to 450°F.

2. In a large bowl toss all ingredients up to the jalapeños with a light coating of olive oil. Season with sea salt. Spread vegetables out on 2 sheet trays, making sure they are in a

single layer. This will ensure proper roasting and caramelization and prevent steaming. Roast vegetables 10-15 minutes; the broccolini will be finished cooking first, check it
after about 9 minutes; use tongs to remove it to a plate and
continue roasting the roots.

3. Toss to ensure even cooking. Roast 15-25 minutes
more or until just cooked firm, but you can pierce the
yams with a fork, and their edges are a bit crispy. Let cool
5 minutes, then transfer to a bowl; toss gently with cilantro
sprigs.

Adapted from Gregory Gourdet.

BEHIND THE LESSONS:

Me

I was nearly finished writing this book. It was a beautiful Sunday in New York City, the sky as bright and clear as I remembered it being a decade prior. The calendar called for quiet reflection, but the weather called for brunch. Mourners were gathered at the newly opened memorial pools where the Twin Towers once stood. For many of us, it was a day for gathering friends around a generous bread-basket and pots of coffee with cream, as a balm to soothe our more generalized sadness and the anxiety that came with the city's heightened state of alert. It was a day for sharing memories, and I was struck by how prominently food figured into many of them, well beyond that child-hood dinner of clams and duck on the hundred-and-seventh floor.

In the months after my arrival from California, when I was barely making rent on a MacDougal Street walk-up, I ate an awful lot of Ray's pizza by the slice, cold sesame noodles from Empire Szechuan, and Macoun apples, which I'd never seen on the West Coast. I started dating a writer I had met while we were both working at *Life* magazine, and as the relationship turned more serious, we pooled our re-sources to celebrate birthdays at stellar restaurants like Gramercy Tavern (with a pre–*Top Chef* Tom Colicchio at the helm). After we had been together for seven (seven!) years, generous friends cheered our engagement with an absurdly luxe caviar-studded dinner at Petrossian on Fifty-

Eighth Street. My last supper before becoming a mother was udon-and-tempura-shrimp soup from the Japanese noodle place around the corner from us, and eight days after my son's birth we showed him off to family and friends over bagels and smoked Gaspe salmon from the Lower East Side's Russ & Daughters.

Life is meals.

I've never looked back at a milestone and thought about how little I ate at the time. Good food is important to me, and more so to chefs. If you're going to reconsider how you eat, chefs will join that conversation with enthusiasm. After nearly a year of listening to dozens of chefs discuss their feelings about food, I had not only learned a lot about how to live a life in healthy balance with what I wanted to eat, but had internalized some very simple and valuable truths:

- Enjoy the food you love.
- Cook most of your meals.
- Eat all of your vegetables.
- Lemon, salt, and olive oil are all you need to make almost any dish terrific.
- Have some fennel.
- Take the doggie bag.
- End your day with a square of chocolate.

Friends (and sometimes strangers who learned about my project) wanted to know: Did I lose weight? Yes! I didn't have loads of weight to lose, but I did shape up while eating and feeding my family really well. I ate out a fair amount, but also cooked more than ever. I even sometimes remembered to pack a lunch, owing in part to the fact that I stopped flailing around in the morning and settled on a rotation of plain Greek yogurt with fruit, oatmeal, or eggs—with or without spinach. Exercise was an important piece of the equation, and I found myself squarely in the camp of those who run the extra mile in order to eat the extra piece of especially great bread, but who practice yoga just because it feels good.

A little coda to my Ferran Adrià story. Two years after that first interview, when he told me you don't read a book about architecture and try to build your own house (and you don't read a book from the world's foremost avant-garde chef and expect to cook like him), I saw the great man again. It was a party for his follow-up tome, which, to my surprise, was comprised of recipes for the home cook with step-by-step photographs and instruction so basic it reminded the reader to have a supply of paper towels in the kitchen. He now had an evangelical fervor to teach regular folk to feed themselves, to eat nourishing home-cooked food, and to enjoy a fruit-based dessert, "for a joyful ending to a meal," most nights. "People have time to cook," Adrià told me. "They spend four hours watching TV! So they have time. You can watch TV *and* cook!"

He's right, of course. Though I still sometimes scramble to get dinner onto the table in the tiny window between the end of my workday and the hour in which I find my child hungry enough to eat his own hand, we sit down together often. My greatest triumph? Dinner is not always pasta. It might be Eric Ripert's toaster-oven paillard or Naomi Pomeroy's tomato soup, or Joe Bastianich's white beans and chard. Or it is something of my own creation, a remix of leftovers and some oddball vegetable. Weekends are for more ambitious fare, or for roasting a chicken, which takes place largely unattended, so I can enjoy my life outside of the kitchen. Will any of these be the meals that my son someday recalls with fondness—our family's future classics? Can anything in my new repertoire rise to the vaunted position of my father's Turkish Pizza-pie Eggs?

So, for my final recipe, an offering from one nonchef. You don't need the training of an architect to replicate it; yet it was an essential ingredient in making our house a home.

Morris Adato's Turkish Pizza-pie Eggs

serves 4

2 tablespoons butter

10 mushrooms, sliced

1 large ripe tomato, roughly chopped

1 teaspoon oregano, or more to taste

9 large eggs, well beaten

2 ounces feta cheese, crumbled (about 1/3 cup,
   loosely packed)

1 ounce Parmesan cheese, grated (about ½ cup,
   loosely packed)

2 ounces Kasseri (or Turkish Kasar) cheese, grated
   (may substitute provolone)

Salt and pepper to taste

1. Warm a large skillet over medium heat and melt a quarter of the butter. Add the sliced mushrooms and sauté until soft and slick. Remove from pan and keep handy.

2. Add remaining butter to pan and melt. Add chopped tomato and press the pieces with the flat of a fork until they break into a mostly liquid sauce, about 3 to 5 minutes. Season with oregano and add the beaten eggs, then the cheeses.

3. Reduce heat to low and stir constantly until eggs are nearly firm, but still moist. Season with salt and pepper to taste (Morris's way: lots of pepper, not much salt—the cheeses are salty on their own.) Stir in sautéed mushrooms and serve at once with toasted onion bialys, brewed decaf, fresh orange juice, and the Sunday paper.

ACKNOWLEDGMENTS

My real and big thanks to…

Art Smith for his inspiration, the foreword, and for Put-Ups Salad.

Tracy Bernstein, my insightful and enthusiastic editor, who noticed before I did that this book was not just about chefs.

Also at NAL: exquisitely careful copy editor Tiffany Yates Martin, and infinitely patient cover designer Monica Benal-cazar.

Caryn Karmatz Rudy, who—hooray!—became my agent before I had the chance to grapple with the fact that she doesn't like butter, cheese, or condiments. (And Todd Shuster for introducing me to Caryn.)

Neeti Madan for early guidance, and notes on the proposal that prefigured this book.

Larry Hackett, Betsy Gleick, Kim Hubbard, Nancy Jeffrey, Tatsha Robertson, Sharon Cotliar, Andy Abrahams, J. D. Heyman, and all my pals at *People* magazine, who allowed me the time for this project and remained supportive throughout.

Great women who helped me navigate chef world: Sarah Abell, Jennifer Baum, Rebecca Brooks, Robin Insley, Becca Parrish, Helen Medvedovsky, Tammy Walker, Willie Norkin and Kim Yorio. Also, Larry Carrino. And Susan Gross for above, beyond, and lunch. (And Lee Schrager for so considerately gathering up so many chefs.)

Opinionated readers and fine travel companions: Jordonna Sabih Grace, Jennifer Markowitz, LeiLani Nishime, Andrea Rosenfeld and Susan Rothwell.

Rebecca Klus, who cheerfully tested and retested recipes and gave good advice. (And Melissa Clark for introducing me to Rebecca.)

Ellen Shapiro, a wise foodie-researcher, who kept me in line factually. Lynn Colomello, who transcribed many of my interviews. (And Maxine Paetro for introducing me to Lynn, plus for long lists of other stuff.)

Photographer Rachel Papo. (And Lisa Robinson and Ken Rosenthal for introducing me to Rachel; also Ken for some other things I'll remember later.)

Lorena Palmer for the constant and seamless help she brings to my family.

Gale Kaufman, Mick, Josh, and Alex van Biema for cheering across rivers.

Michael Adato, who has come around on the subject of clams if not neckties, for his quiet encouragement.

Sharon and Morris for support and love that crosses continents. You still feed me.

Recipe Index

Halibut
   Ceviche with jalapeño and parsley 276
   "Gyros" 236
Maine Lobster 152
Paella, with chicken 280
Salmon
   Provençal, with tomato-basil sauce 13
   Seared, with lentils 115
Scoglio (seafood pasta) 48
Shrimp burgers 185
Sturgeon wrapped in prosciutto 114

MEAT
   Pork fried rice 243
   Shredded beef, Mexican 85
   Steak with horseradish dressing 184

SOUP
   Chicken and dumplings 206
   Creamy Asian tomato 90
   Hangover soup 183
   Kombu and chickpea, with Tuscan kale 262

SWEETS
   Apple Galette 172
   Chocolate-covered cereal 169
   Lemon-almond cookies 170
   Spice-roasted stone fruit 173

VEGETARIAN DISHES
   Beet sandwiches with avocado, grapefruit, and radish sprouts 133
   Bulgur with sun-dried tomatoes, raisins, pine nuts, and olives 259
   Grilled vegetable tacos 87
   Pea salad with basil and pea shoots 240
   Quinoa with summer vegetables 239
   Roasted vegetables with olive oil, ginger, and chili 282
   Spaghetti pomodoro 46
   Spring vegetable salad 151
   Summer succotash 152
   Warm asparagus salad with soft-boiled eggs 32
   Watermelon and tomato salad with feta and olives 91
   White bean stew with Swiss chard and tomatoes 208
   Yountville three bean salad 29